Praise for

No More Knee Pain

"*No More Knee Pain* is a must-read for any woman who has or wants to avoid knee problems. Dr. Kessler explores the conventional orthopedic approach, as well as the holistic approach. The reader will soon realize that one treatment form is not better than the other, but synergistic. After reading this book, the reader will be better educated as to the treatment options and outcomes for knee injuries."

—Orrin Sherman, M.D., chief of sports medicine,
New York University and Hospital for Joint Diseases

"*No More Knee Pain* is the first book that describes the association between chronic knee pain and more profound imbalances in the body, mind, and spirit. Dr. Kessler illustrates how stress, nutritional deficiencies, increased inflammation, and hormone imbalances contribute to pain and disability. *No More Knee Pain* offers practical and easy-to-understand guidelines that help restore balance and alleviate pain. This is a truly unique, effective, and holistic approach to this increasingly common chronic condition."

—Allan Warshowsky, M.D.,
director of holistic women's health at the Continuum Center for
Health & Healing, Beth Israel Medical Center,
and author of *Healing Fibroids*

"Dr. George Kessler has written an informative, practical guide that is destined to help the millions afflicted with knee pain."

—Mitchell Gaynor, M.D.,
president and founder of Gaynor Integrative Oncology,
and author of *The Healing Power of Sound*

"In *No More Knee Pain*, women receive an excellent basic guide to natural prevention and relief of knee pain . . . osteopathic physician George Kessler covers all the bases."   —*Midwest Book Review*

"Dr. George Kessler has been able to help many women find relief from pain and, in some cases, reverse the degenerative process—without surgery. He explains how in *No More Knee Pain*."   —*The Oak Ridger*

NO MORE KNEE
PAIN

A WOMAN'S GUIDE TO
NATURAL PREVENTION
AND RELIEF

DR. GEORGE J. KESSLER

with Colleen Kapklein

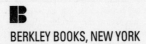

BERKLEY BOOKS, NEW YORK

THE BERKLEY PUBLISHING GROUP
Published by the Penguin Group
Penguin Group (USA) Inc.
375 Hudson Street, New York, New York 10014, USA
Penguin Group (Canada), 90 Eglinton Avenue East, Suite 700, Toronto, Ontario M4P 2Y3, Canada
(a division of Pearson Penguin Canada Inc.)
Penguin Books Ltd., 80 Strand, London WC2R 0RL, England
Penguin Group Ireland, 25 St. Stephen's Green, Dublin 2, Ireland (a division of Penguin Books Ltd.)
Penguin Group (Australia), 250 Camberwell Road, Camberwell, Victoria 3124, Australia
(a division of Pearson Australia Group Pty. Ltd.)
Penguin Books India Pvt. Ltd., 11 Community Centre, Panchsheel Park, New Delhi—110 017, India
Penguin Group (NZ), Cnr. Airborne and Rosedale Roads, Albany, Auckland 1310, New Zealand
(a division of Pearson New Zealand Ltd.)
Penguin Books (South Africa) (Pty.) Ltd., 24 Sturdee Avenue, Rosebank, Johannesburg 2196,
South Africa

Penguin Books Ltd., Registered Offices: 80 Strand, London WC2R 0RL, England

Interior art provided by: Nucleus Medical Art, www.nucleusinc.com; Saunders' Exercise Xpress, The
Saunders Group, Inc.; PhysioTools, Peter Konrad, Fitness and Sports Therapy; and PhysioTools,
Christopher M. Norris, Weight Training.
Cover design by Rita Frangie.

PRINTING HISTORY
Berkley hardcover edition / April 2004
Berkley trade paperback edition / December 2005

Berkley trade paperback ISBN: 0-425-20694-7

The Library of Congress has cataloged the Berkley hardcover edition as follows:

Kessler, George J.
    No more knee pain / George J. Kessler with Colleen Kapklein.—1st ed.
      p.   cm.
    Includes index.
    ISBN 0-425-19400-0
    1. Knee—Diseases—Treatment—Popular works. 2. Knee—Wounds and injuries—
treatment—Popular works. 3. Pain—Treatment—Popular works. 4. Pain—Alternative
treatment—Popular works. 5. Women—Diseases—Treatment—Popular works. I.
Kapklein, Colleen. II. Title.

RC951.K476 2004
617.5'82—dc22

                                                                    2004041001

PRINTED IN THE UNITED STATES OF AMERICA

10 9 8 7 6 5 4 3 2 1

PUBLISHER'S NOTE: Every effort has been made to ensure that the information contained in this
book is complete and accurate. However, neither the publisher nor the author is engaged in rendering
professional advice or services to the individual reader. The ideas, procedures, and suggestions contained in this book are not intended as a substitute for consulting with your physician. All matters regarding your health require medical supervision. Neither the author nor the publisher shall be liable or
responsible for any loss or damage allegedly arising from any information or suggestion in this book.
The publisher does not have any control over and does not assume any responsibility for author or third-
party websites or their content.

To my wife and partner, Linda Diane Weiss Kessler

In loving memory of Betty Jean Bremner Lysohir, 1927–2003

CONTENTS

Acknowledgments

I would like to acknowledge and give thanks to many people without whom this book would not have been written.

I give special thanks to my wonderful and loving children, Emily and Katie, who make my life complete.

Colleen Kapklein, a true collaborative partner, who made the process of organizing and writing this book a joyful adventure.

Janis Vallely, my agent and friend, whose belief in me and efforts on my behalf are truly appreciated.

Meredith Bernstein, the Putnam Berkley Group, and especially my editor, Denise Silvestro, for her kindness, wisdom and support.

My office staff—Brenda Hughes, Denise Tirado, Tamika Salter and Melissa Bernal—for creating the environment that makes my practice so wonderful to be in.

Special thanks to Dr. Robert Kessler, Dr. Michael Konig, Dr. Sun Fook Ka, Russell Hartophilis, R. P. T., Dr. Michael Borkin, Dr. Orrin Sherman, and the members of the Anne L. Wales, D.O., Study Group, who always remind me that the smallest unit we can treat is the whole.

To my many friends, too numerous to mention, who have contributed insight into this process.

I would like to conclude with a most sincere and heartfelt thanks to my patients, who continue to inspire and educate me.

INTRODUCTION

No matter how long I practice medicine, I'm still struck daily by the wonder of the human body. Every day I see how things can go wrong, but I am also privileged to witness, over and over again, how nature has created systems of healing. No machine takes care of itself the way the human body can and does.

In this book, I'm addressing the knees specifically, and when you pay attention to them, you can find a whole world there. But this book isn't about—could never be about—"just" the knees. Like any bodily system you might choose to focus on, the knees are a window to the whole body. Every cell in our body has the same genetic information. For the body to function as a whole, every cell has to speak to every other cell every second of the day. So when your knee hurts, it's telling you not only that there may be a mechanical problem in one particular joint but also that something in your body's whole system may require your attention.

No knee is an island. By its very definition as a joint, it connects things. It cannot be considered on its own. To understand what's going wrong in your knee—and how to right it—you have to look at the knee in the context of the whole body. Furthermore, you have to look at the health of the whole body holistically.

And so we must ask, when our knees are failing us, if the point is really that we are failing our knees.

Right now, our society is losing the war on chronic diseases; we're getting more and more of them, at younger and younger ages. In large part, that's because our medical system is devoted to "curing" very specific sets of symptoms while overlooking the underlying problems causing those symptoms. Nature has struck a delicate balance within our bodies, and when we fall out of balance, we run into trouble. When we focus on re-creating that natural balance, viewing our bodies as wholes greater than the sum of their parts, we lead ourselves toward a path of wellness.

Conventional medicine by itself is going to get you only so far. The failure of modern medicine is that it looks at people only when they are sick, and then only as having gotten a disease that must be diagnosed and treated (and it isn't a disease until an insurance code can be found that matches up with it!). You might get a thyroid diagnosis from your endocrinologist, a bowel diagnosis from your gastroenterologist, and a skin diagnosis from your dermatologist. If you ask each specialist if the problems are related, they will (most likely) say no. But how can they not be? They are all happening within the same package, through all the same systems, and in cells with the same genetic information.

As a system of specialists oriented toward addressing disease and injury with drugs and surgery, mainstream contemporary medicine is very, very good at what it does. If I get shot, by all means take me immediately to the nearest trauma center. But what it does takes you only up to a certain point. Now if you've torn this or sprained that and you know the moment of injury, conventional medicine may be all you need. Go under the knife, do so many weeks of rehab, and you'll be good to go. But if your issue is less clearly defined, if your problem is more chronic, if the usual treatments don't resolve your trouble, you need the whole-body, whole-life approach of integrative medicine—the best that all high-tech conventional medicine has to offer *and* the insights of the best proven "alternative" or "complementary" methods. In most cases, natural, noninvasive techniques will be all you need to get you, quite literally, back on your feet—pain-free.

Most people don't have disease, they have dis-ease, or breakdowns in balanced bodily function. The symptoms we suffer are a result of that imbalance. Symptoms in the knee are no different. Most are not caused by disease but by disturbances of proper functioning. For example, if you don't drink enough water over a long period of time, dehydration will not only make your lips and tongue dry but also the cartilage in your knees. Your shock absorbers won't work well, and you will have pain with certain activities. As another example, if your muscles are weak for any reason, they won't be able to balance or support your joints in motion, and you'll have poor mechanical use of your knee, resulting in knee pain. A hormonal shift might also create an imbalance that can lead to (among other things) knee pain, as can a seemingly unrelated illness, as Susan's story, on the next page, illustrates.

Susan

Susan never gave a thought to her knees until one day when she was fifty-two and, as she says, menopause "crashed down" on her. "When I woke up in the morning feeling like an eighteen-wheeler had run over my body and left its tire tracks on me in my sleep, I wished my body belonged to somebody else," she told me. "I was stiff, stiff, stiff. I felt like I did not have the energy to drag myself out of bed. Climbing stairs was like punishment. Trying to lift my knees felt like lifting lead weights. At the end of the day, when I was tired, I had to use my hands on the handrail to pull myself up the last three steps of the flight just to get up to my bedroom."

All this from a woman who had once danced professionally. Susan hadn't taken up belly dancing until her early thirties and had initially gone into it primarily for the exercise. But soon she had found an unusual passion for the movement. It seemed ironic now, but her specialty had once been a dance done on her knees, featuring a series of ripples and shimmies that whirled her around until she was kneeling, after which she would intricately dance her way back up again. Making it look easy and natural was part of the challenge.

Susan quit dancing when her day job got demanding, and she devoted all of her time to climbing the corporate ladder. Unfortunately, that meant she stopped exercising altogether. But the lack never seemed to cause her any problems—until menopause hit and her joints started to hurt, especially her knees. Now the woman in my office moved like someone much older, and her dancer's grace was nothing but a memory thanks to sore knees.

She'd learned from friends about glucosamine and chondroitin, MSM, and arnica ointment, and at another friend's insistence, she'd started exercising again too, a gentle workout guided by a morning television show. With all that in place, she began to feel better. Then, in routine screening, her internist discovered she was having bone loss, and Susan feared she'd get worse again. In addition, she developed arthritis in her fingers. Memories of her grandmother—living with crippling arthritis into her nineties, ultimately holding her spoon in a fist, the way children do—haunted Susan. That's when she came to see me.

I told Susan I thought she was already doing some very important things to care for her knees. I did suggest a bit of fine-tuning: adding bromelain and horse chestnut, and increasing the amount of exercise she was getting with some weight training. She noticed increased flexibility almost immediately, in her knees as well as her fingers, and she described her joints as feeling "lighter."

Still, though some symptoms were abating, I wanted to pinpoint the ultimate cause of those symptoms and eliminate that if we could. Tests for thyroid antibodies turned up positive, and after some searching we discovered the culprit: Susan had a parasite infection from years ago. She'd been entirely unaware of it after an initial illness, which (she thought) cleared up quickly, though looking back she could trace a long chain of symptoms back to it. It turned out that many of those nagging complaints, which she had either considered unrelated or blamed on menopause, were the result of a protracted immune battle.

With a course of antibiotics supported by an excellent diet, the elimination of foods she was sensitive to, and some supplements, we got rid of the parasite, and an array of symptoms cleared up—primary among them her joint pain. (And she now tested negative for thyroid antibodies.)

Six years later, Susan still follows the insulin resistance–type diet described later in this book and takes a few supplements, and her knees remain pain-free. Now some days she slips on her old leotards and skirts, flips on the music and belly dances around her living room. She might not make those elaborate knee landings anymore, but she's still got quite a repertoire of arches, contractions and figure eights. And she does a mean shimmy.

I see women like Susan in my practice every day. Joint pain is one of the most common complaints I hear. Most people get joint pains as they get older, although I hear about knee pain from every age group. In my practice, the vast majority of menopausal women tell me their joints hurt, and an extremely large percentage of those women focus on their knees. I treat both men and women for knee pain, of course, but most women I see have knee pain with no history of injury, while men are more likely to come in after a specific trauma to the knee. It is often easier to get satisfactory treatment for knee pain resulting from some kind of immediate trauma—it's just the kind of thing contemporary mainstream medicine is good at. Yet many of my patients have sought help from a variety of doctors but found little relief. Although knee pain arises from a wide range of causes, only one of which is osteoarthritis, fortunately most of these patients have something in common with Susan: the ability to make that pain go away—without surgery and without a lifetime of powerful pharmaceuticals. This book shows that you can have that ability too.

Women and Knee Pain

Knee pain affects many millions of Americans each year, the majority of them women. Government statistics show knee pain is about three times as prevalent in women over sixty as in men of that age. Approximately one in four women overall have daily knee pain, and the figure is even higher in Hispanic and African-American women. There's no magic age at which knees become a problem, though the incidence of knee pain increases with age, stepping up particularly around menopause. Baby boom women have more than a passing familiarity with knee pain; if they don't suffer from it themselves, the odds are they know someone who does. Younger women don't escape, however, and many have undefined knee pain (not caused by injury), perhaps connected to hormonal imbalance, body alignment problems, or even ordinary life stresses such as too much work, too little sleep, and caring for everyone but themselves. Even young girls are increasingly contending with knee injuries, usually from sports. Injuries are on the rise for women of all ages, as our essentially sedentary lifestyles clash with our "weekend warrior" approach to exercise. While we rack up enough birthdays to cause seemingly inevitable wear and tear on our joints, knee pain sends eleven million Americans to doctors' offices each year. That's not counting all the people who don't seek treatment even for chronic and sometimes severe knee pain. And since women are more likely to have chronic, poorly defined knee pain (compared to men, who are more likely to have pain related to an obvious injury), the bulk of those suffering in silence are surely women.

In one major study, the more knee pain patients reported, the more difficulty the subjects had with even basic physical functions, to the point where their quality of life was definitely affected. We're talking about chronic knee pain that is far more than the occasional twinge or a minor annoyance. We're talking about pain that changes your life. And, in this book, we're talking about how to change it back. We tend to accept knee pain, and osteoarthritis, as normal parts of aging. But they don't have to be!

Over two million people have knee surgery every year in this country. Women are more likely than men to need complete knee replacement. Those going under the knife for any knee-related reason are probably also disproportionately female, because in addition to being more prone to arthritis than men, women are also more susceptible to knee injuries. Women suffer many sports injuries more frequently than men, and women are more likely to get injured even in noncontact sports. For instance, women participating in sports that involve a lot of jumping and pivoting, such as basketball and tennis (or even step aerobics classes), are between two and eight times more likely than men to tear a certain ligament (ACL). Women are at greater risk of injuring the kneecap than are men. They are far more likely to develop "runner's knee." And on and on.

Of course, it isn't just injuries causing women knee pain. For one thing, even well-healed injuries can increase the risk of getting osteoarthritis down the line. In addition, various reports show that fully 12 percent of adults over 25 have symptomatic arthritis (with rates rising up to 1 in 5 with age). Those thirty-three million people (minimum) are disproportionately female, as osteoarthritis is far more common in women than in men. And in women with osteoarthritis, the knee is the joint most commonly affected.

Pain in general affects women differently than it does men. With ninety million people in this country living with chronic pain, it pays to try to untangle the differences. For starters, women are more likely to feel pain: A Gallup poll shows that 46 percent of women have pain of some type daily, whereas only 37 percent of men report a similar experience. Pain also seems to have a bigger impact on daily life in women, who are 50 percent more likely than men to miss work because of pain, to take just one example.

To complicate matters, women and men may experience different symptoms as a result of similar causes. For example, a man with the same kneecap or cartilage issue as a woman may not feel the pain as acutely since larger muscle mass (which men, on average, have) can protect against or diminish some problems. To take another example, depression may not manifest outside of mood changes in one person, while in another, the chain reaction may include knee pain.

Furthermore, treatments may affect women differently. To take just one basic example, over-the-counter pain relievers help women less than they do men. Many treatments that work for men may not work for women, or at least not as well. The same is true in reverse, but the fact remains that much of mainstream medicine has been studied only in men. (Ironically, that's because researchers fear women's shifting hormones could confuse results, a tacit acknowledgment that these things do work differently in male and female bodies.) Even after almost a decade of federal law stating that women must be included in research, the *New York Times* reported on three different studies showing that researchers often ignore the mandate or don't analyze the data they collect to address it. Women are also more likely to benefit from "alternative" and mind-body treatments—and, not coincidentally, I'm sure, more likely to seek them out.

Whatever the source, far too many women live with chronic knee pain that either hasn't been properly diagnosed or hasn't responded well to conventional treatments. They face a medical world too ready to dismiss their complaints as "all in your head"—a "diagnosis" handed down disproportionately to women—and more likely to treat men with similar symptoms. Many doctors also use a working model that assumes women are essentially scale models of men. Well, they are not. Women's unique anatomical and physiological makeup determines when and how their knees fail—and, more importantly, how to get and keep them strong and healthy.

That's why this book outlines a brand-new program designed especially for women that will have you feeling better—stronger, healthier, and in much less pain—within six weeks, and pain-free and better than ever within twelve. Without drugs. Without surgery. *With* diet, nutritional supplements, and the right exercises, within a holistic framework that considers all the interlocking systems in your body as well as your mental and emotional health. It's the program that's worked for dozens, if not hundreds, of women in my practice. It has turned around many, many cases of severe, chronic pain from a variety of causes, but it also eliminates the knee pain familiar to just about everyone over forty: stiff knees when you stand up at the end of a movie, achy knees after driving a car with the seat imperfectly adjusted, sore knees after a good workout, pain in the morning or when it is stormy.

Mainstream Medicine

Before we go any further, I do want to point out that I am not entirely against surgery and good drugs. In the right time and place, they are awesome and effective tools. I sometimes recommend them myself. The problem is, they are doled out too early, too easily and too often— and often when they will be inadequate anyway. If you've torn a ligament and need to get back on the court as soon as possible, you may well need a surgical repair. But surgery doesn't usually fix the problem that brought about your knee damage in the first place, and if you don't address the underlying cause, given enough time you're just going to end up needing a second round of surgery. (And if you're going to go after those root causes anyway, you might as well do it before surgery—and find out if that treatment is sufficient on its own.) If that's not enough to make you think twice, consider this: One common knee surgery often ends up being "diagnostic"—that is, they go in there, take a look around, see what the problem is and discover they can't really do anything to fix it. And while knee surgery has an excellent chance of resolving your immediate pain crisis, knee surgery has occasionally been associated with chronic knee pain over the long haul. And then there's always the fact that many surgeries simply fail. Even when they do work to solve the immediate crisis, surgery can't reverse degenerative processes—which is just what the program in this book *can* help you do.

Anti-inflammatories such as ibuprofen and some prescription medicines can be a godsend in the face of immediate or chronic pain. But they can cause a host of negative side effects—including gastric ulcers and kidney damage, as well as the more common upset stomach—in many, many users. Besides, taking them may only mask the symptoms, and will never do anything to improve the underlying cause of them. Furthermore, regarding both surgery and drugs, you have to remember that most medical research to date has focused on men—and that women may experience different symptoms for similar ailments and respond differently to the same treatment.

There's a third most common mainstream medicine approach to

knee pain, right up there with cutting and drugging, and this one is particularly familiar to women: the old "there's nothing we can do." Learn to live with it. Grin and bear it. Sometimes this means there is no surgery or drug that addresses your specific problem. Sometimes it means the available diagnostic tests can't pick up your problem. Sometimes it means they just can't find the source of your pain. And sometimes the meta-message is: "There is nothing wrong with your knee." Which is just a heartbeat from "It's all in your head."

This is obviously problematic, and especially so for women. First of all, why should any woman tolerate pain unnecessarily? In almost every case, there *is* something to be done—it's just that it probably wasn't specifically covered in medical school. (Medical students have studied every component of the knee, but they are unlikely to have worked as long and hard on connecting the dots between them to see not only the knee as a whole but also the knee in the context of the whole body.)

Secondly, mainstream medicine historically has a poor track record, too often ignoring women's symptoms when the same complaints in men would receive more aggressive investigation and intervention. We know now that women experience pain more often than men, and are more likely to seek treatment for it—and seek it earlier and more aggressively. Women have lower pain thresholds and less pain tolerance— women, in short, feel more pain. Studies show, for example, that women report more intense pain than do men with the same degree of injury. However, women are better at coping with pain than men, admit to and discuss it more readily than men, and make more effective use of a wider variety of approaches.

Finally, even when something isn't entirely explained by physical findings—that is, when it has psychological, emotional, or even spiritual components (which, in point of fact, almost all physical symptoms do, to some extent)—we should not shrug it off! Rather, we should approach those non-concrete aspects on their own terms and embrace them for what we can learn from them. If they are sometimes a source of the problem, they are also sometimes a source for a solution. There may be nothing your doctor can do for you, but there is most definitely something *you* can do for yourself.

Bringing Me to My Knees

I wrote this book, then, to address all the somethings we *can* do. As it happens, I've got some personal experience with many of them—not just in using them with my patients in my practice but in healing my own knee. I am not a woman, of course, but what I experienced was just the sort of complex interaction of physical and emotional stress that affects so many women—and eludes so many health-care practitioners.

Not long ago I was out jogging as I always do, not particularly hard or fast, and I felt something go wrong. I knew nothing drastic had snapped or broken, but it was bad enough that I had to stop running and go home. This happened at a time of great stress in my life. Not any one major stress, just the accumulation of the pressures of ordinary modern life. I had too many projects going on at once; my office was incredibly busy; my family was in a bit of turmoil over some mountain of a molehill.

At first I just took several days off from running, took some anti-inflammatory herbs, had a couple acupuncture sessions. By the end of the week I felt better, so I went jogging again over the weekend. For less than a quarter of a mile. I knew right away something was still wrong. I'd calmed the most aggressive symptoms, but the underlying cause, whatever it was, was still there.

So I went for physical therapy (to my good friend Russell Hartophilis). Over the course of twelve weeks, doing specific exercises under supervision, I worked back up to being able to run without pain for three miles on the treadmill. That's when I decided I was ready to go back to running outdoors.

In my inaugural run, I pulled my hamstring on the other leg. Clearly, my body still wasn't ready for prime time. So I went back indoors for another three months of PT, and Russell designed an intense full-body workout for me to do at my regular gym. This time around, however, I started to pay attention to the stress I finally realized played a starring role in my little drama. So at the end of each session, I added meditation and Reiki (a kind of energy healing). I also consulted a spiritual healer who works in my office. I reviewed my priorities, and juggled some of my projects to make a bit of breathing space for myself.

Finally, six months after I first hurt myself, I was really and truly ready to be on my own—ready physically, but also mentally and emotionally. I could be independent of my physical therapist—and independent of pain. I successfully resumed my regular jogging routine, pain-free.

The Body-Mind-*Knee* Connection

This whole episode brought home to me like never before the message I'm always emphasizing to the women I counsel about knee pain: When it comes to health, you have to consider the whole person—body, mind and spirit. You can't just treat one symptom and expect a cure. You might temporarily alleviate whatever is bothering you that way, but you will never get to the real source of the problem and you'll constantly be open to recurrence—or something worse. In the fine tradition of teaching what you need to learn, I had ignored the true message my body was sending, and earned myself an additional injury and double the recovery time in the process. My knee pain was an SOS signal I didn't acknowledge at first. It wasn't until I took it seriously and did what I had to do to effect a rescue—and until I decided to let this program work for me—that I put my knee pain behind me. Neither PT nor meditation and stress reduction alone could have done the trick. Yes, my injury—a physical response—had physical repercussions. The pain sent signals to the muscles, which got progressively weaker. I had to strengthen them again. But doing that alone was, as I found out the hard way, a short-term solution at best (about one quarter of a mile's worth, to be exact). Focusing initially only on muscle strength was just ineffective. I needed to treat my body, mind and soul.

Fortunately, you can do it right the first time. That's where the program laid out in this book comes in. The book begins by giving you some background: a look at the healthy knee, then at what goes wrong and how and where. I'll also discuss the unique aspects of women's knees, and how those differences affect diagnosis and treatment of knee pain. After reviewing what mainstream medicine offers women and how to know when and if it will help you, I'll lay out my plan for healthy, pain-free knees, centered on nutrition, exercise, posture, and stress reduction (both physical and psychological), backed up by natural, holistic remedies and spiritual development. I'll tell you the foods you need to eat and those to avoid; the ways of moving your body that help and harm your knees; the exercises that strengthen or stress your muscles and joints; and the mental, emotional and even spiritual paths that help or hinder your healing.

The knee is the biggest joint in the body, and it connects the two longest bones. So if you were taking the design specs back to the drawing board, you might aim for a sturdier model. Unfortunately, we're stuck with the only knees we'll ever have (barring those who get surgical replacements), so we need to take care of them. That's why this plan is as much for prevention as for healing. The best way to have pain-free knees is to keep them in their natural state from the beginning. If it is already too late for that, the program in this book will also help you regain healthy knees. The fate of any given pair of knees depends on that person's unique genetics, biochemistry, environment, body mechanics and general state of being; but no matter what factors have influenced your particular knees, the program in this book can strengthen them and prevent and even reverse knee pain.

Along the way, I'll answer important, overlooked and sometimes surprising questions about knee pain—everything from why your knee pain seems worse at certain points in your menstrual cycle, why your knee is stiff and painful with weather changes, and why you get muscle weakness around the knee, to how low thyroid hormone levels contribute to knee pain, how depression can damage your knees (and how knee pain can depress you), and how sugar impacts your knees, as well as the connections between sleep, stress, spirituality, anorexia, meditation and your knees.

The facts have the potential to revolutionize your life. If dealing with knee pain limits you in any way, know you don't have to just accept the notion that your pain will be with you for the rest of your days. The straightforward strategies here can help you make knee pain a thing of the past.

1

What's in a Knee?

You really need your knees. You not only need knees in order to bend and straighten your leg, but you'd be hard-pressed to move around without these simple hinges: They are what allow you to sit, stand, walk, jump and pivot. Knees are anatomical shock-absorbers, and they allow you to balance and to adjust your center of gravity. They quite literally support you in your life, and help you move forward in the world. Before we get to how to protect your knees and keep them healthy for a lifetime, this chapter will help you understand the structure and function of healthy knees, and the most common things that go wrong with them. Once we've covered the things all knees have in common, we'll take a look at what is unique about women's knees, and why they need special attention.

The knee is the biggest joint in the body, and it connects the two longest bones (thigh and shin). Yet for all that, it isn't all that sturdy. Ball-and-socket joints—like the one at your hip—are more secure than a hinge like the knee. Instead of fitting into each other like the bones in a ball-and-socket joint, the bones in the knee look more like a teacup (the rounded base of the thigh bone) resting on a saucer (the top of the shin bone). The knee is made up of bones, cartilage, muscles, ligaments, tendons and soft tissues.

Bones

Three bones come together at the knee: the upper thigh bone (femur), which connects the pelvis to the knee; the shin bone (tibia), which connects the ankle to the knee; and the kneecap (patella). (In addition, the fibula, in the lower leg, though technically not the knee, is also important, as it holds and stabilizes the tibia.) The patella is about two-by-three inches to three-by-four inches. It covers, or caps, the other bones at the front of the knee, and works both to protect the joint and to give the muscles leverage. It slides over a groove in the thigh bone when the leg moves.

Cartilage

This tough yet flexible, jelly-like and elastic connective tissue covers and cushions the ends of bones, including the three in the knee, to help absorb shocks from weight above and to keep the knee from being jarred from below. It seems almost painted on the bone. Cartilage holds water, so it can slide easily and let the bones glide over one another so the joints move smoothly.

You'll be hearing a lot more about the circular pads of cartilage known as menisci, in particular. Located between the thigh and shin bones on both sides (outer and inner) of each knee, the menisci provide stability, keep the bones from moving side to side, and distribute

FRONT VIEW

BACK VIEW

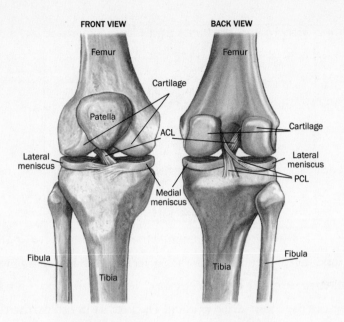

Femur

Cartilage

Patella

ACL

Lateral meniscus

Medial meniscus

Fibula

Tibia

Femur

Cartilage

Lateral meniscus

PCL

Tibia

Fibula

OUTSIDE (LATERAL) VIEW

INSIDE (MEDIAL) VIEW

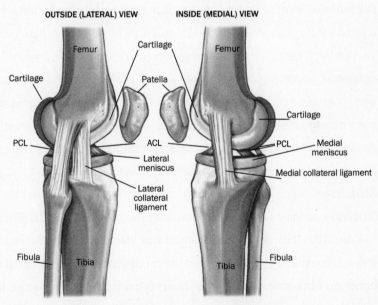

Femur

Cartilage

Patella

Cartilage

PCL

ACL

Lateral meniscus

Lateral collateral ligament

Fibula

Tibia

Femur

Cartilage

PCL

Medial meniscus

Medial collateral ligament

Tibia

Fibula

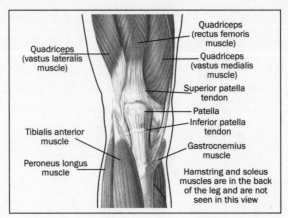

Quadriceps
(vastus lateralis
muscle)

Quadriceps
(rectus femoris
muscle)

Quadriceps
(vastus medialis
muscle)

Superior patella
tendon

Patella

Inferior patella
tendon

Tibialis anterior
muscle

Peroneus longus
muscle

Gastrocnemius
muscle

Hamstring and soleus
muscles are in the back
of the leg and are not
seen in this view

weight more evenly, cushioning the lower part of the leg against the weight of the rest of the body.

When cartilage gets dried out and cracked, as in osteoarthritis, the parts of the joints can no longer glide past each other as they were designed to do, and swelling, pain and inhibited movement can result. Fortunately, cartilage is reparable, via nutrients coupled with the elimination of harmful physical stress—and that's just what this book sets out to guide you in. (If your case is advanced to the degree that you have changes in your bones themselves, I still think the method described will work, though it hasn't been suitably studied yet.)

Muscles

The knee contains two main groups of muscles: the quadriceps and the hamstrings. The four quadriceps muscles on the front of the thigh straighten the leg, while the hamstrings, on the back of the thigh, bend it. Their opposing forces lend dynamic strength to the knee. In addition, the gastroc-soleus group—the calf muscles—while not in the knee itself, directly affects the knee.

Ligaments

Very strong and just a little bit flexible, ligaments are tough bands of tissue that connect bones to each other. They hold the knee (as well as other joints) together. Ligaments stabilize the knee, making sure bones stay within their expected range of motion. Without them, you wouldn't be able to walk, run, or do much of anything else that involves moving the knee in the slightest.

There are four main ligaments connecting the thigh and shin bones in the knee, stabilizing the joint and holding the leg bones together so you can move. You have two collateral ligaments, the medial collateral ligament (MCL) on the inner side of the knee and the lateral collateral ligament (LCL) on the outer side. You also have the cruciate ligaments in the center of the knee: the anterior cruciate ligament (ACL)—a very popular one to injure—which connects the back of the thigh bone to the front of the shin bone, and the posterior cruciate ligament (PCL). The collateral ligaments connect the upper and lower bones and prevent side to side movement. The cruciate ligaments keep the knee from overextending or over-rotating.

Tendons

Tendons are tough, fibrous cords or bands that extend from muscle tissues to provide a strong attachment to bones. We tend to talk about tendons and muscles as separate things, but in reality muscle becomes tendon as it approaches the bone. There is a long transition zone in which the fibers of each intermingle as muscle changes to tendon.

Tendons contain Golgi fiber apparatus, a type of nerve fiber. The Golgi fibers register the amount of tension placed on them by the muscles and communicate this information to the brain, which sends back instructions for the muscles to follow. This allows muscles to lengthen and shorten to accommodate the demands on them. The Golgi fiber can also turn the muscle off and on in response to pain, and make and relieve spasms. Part of what physical therapy does is change the communication between the brain and the muscles via these Golgi bodies; this can reestablish normal signals to and from the muscles, thereby changing the length and function of the muscles toward normal.

The main tendon in the knee is the quadriceps tendon, which connects the muscles of the same name to the kneecap and the lower leg, providing the power to extend the leg. The patellar tendon connects the kneecap and the shinbone, so it is really a ligament, but given its common name I'm including it here. The patella is actually located within the tendon, and the tendon continues on to attach to the bone.

It is just as important to understand how the knee fits into the whole body as it is to understand how the different parts of the knee work together, and we'll get to that later in the book. For now, just remember that by its very definition as a joint, the knee connects different parts of the body.

What Goes Wrong

"Problem" knees generally result from injury, simple wear and tear, overuse or misuse. Over time, this can result in arthritis. Athletes are especially prone to this, but knee pain is most definitely an equal opportunity offender, and all kinds of people can have problem knees.

No matter what your specific diagnosis—or lack thereof—the underlying cause of symptoms is almost always inflammation and its telltale signs of redness, heat, swelling and pain, and even diminished or sometimes lost function (not necessarily all at once). Inflammation is a normal process—it's the way the body fixes tissues and defends against infection. But the inflammatory response can be excessive, and when it is, it's a problem.

ARTHRITIS OF THE KNEE

We'll start with what is, along with strain from injury, the most common knee complaint. "Arthritis" can mean any one of over one hundred joint conditions, but most often when you hear about arthritis of the knee, what is being referred to is osteoarthritis (OA). Osteoarthritis is a degenerative condition in which cartilage gradually wears away, leaving the bones unprotected. Instead of gliding over each other at the joint, the bone surfaces rub against each other painfully. (Rheumatoid arthritis, an autoimmune disease, also affects the joints, including the knee, as the joint becomes inflamed and the cartilage gets destroyed, but this is a separate and somewhat less common condition.) OA is bad enough by itself, with your knee stressed and inflamed, but it also leaves you more prone to injury. The relationship goes the other way around too, with injuries making you more prone to arthritis.

Your body is constantly both building up and breaking down cartilage, and OA occurs when the breakdown part of the cycle gets out of hand. When you first get cartilage damage, your body simply builds new cartilage, and this can keep your knee working well for years. The reconstruction can't keep up with the demolition indefinitely, however, and in the end the breakdown outpaces the buildup, causing pain and loss of function in the joint.

Osteoarthritis begins with loss of fluid from the cartilage (water being a main component of cartilage). When the cartilage dries out and gets cracked, resulting in irritation of the bones under the cracks, the bone tries to relieve the irritation, creating new calcification—new bone—which results in calcium deposits where they don't belong. That's what is seen on an X ray when your doctors says, "It's arthritis." But the process is underway long before you can see such bony changes. Your doctor may say there's "nothing" in the X ray, but your pain is signaling that the process has begun—it just hasn't proceeded far enough to show up on an X ray. Even an MRI may not show it, though the machine can be set up to focus specifically on checking cartilage, which may be worth a try. But even if nothing shows up, just because you don't meet the diagnostic criteria of mainstream medicine doesn't mean you don't have the process that leads to OA going on. Don't settle for being told there's nothing there when your pain is telling you otherwise. In fact, it is far better and easier to reverse the process before bone damage has occurred.

While the mechanism of OA is reasonably clear, the precise cause of osteoarthritis is more muddled. We do know that osteoarthritis occurs in an overstressed joint, whether from injury, unfortunate anatomy, or being overweight. In about half the cases, genetics plays a major role in who gets osteoarthritis and who doesn't. Some evidence suggests osteoarthritis may be a whole-body cartilage disease. Despite its reputation as "wear and tear" arthritis, OA often develops simultaneously in different joints, even when you wouldn't expect them to have the same amount of wear and tear, as when both knees develop it although only one sustained an injury, or when joints in the hand start to act up at the same time as the knee.

Whatever the ultimate cause, the knee is the most common joint affected by osteoarthritis, and even more significantly so in women than in men. That's on top of the fact that osteoarthritis itself is more common in women and, for unknown reasons, more common still in African-American women, who also tend to get it younger than other women or men. In women, OA often appears in both knees and tends to be associated with being overweight (compared to men who more often get OA connected to an old injury, and therefore often only on one side). Osteoarthritis is most common in middle-aged and older people, though it is showing up at younger and younger ages, with rates increasing steadily with age, especially after about thirty-five to fifty years old. Older women are twice as likely to have OA than women twenty years their junior. Younger people with arthritis tend to have their genes, or an old injury, to thank for it. But osteoarthritis *should not be* an inevitable part of getting older, and this book will show you how to write it right out of the script of your life.

Although you can have OA without having symptoms, knees with arthritis generally feel painful and stiff, and may become knobby or bony or enlarged or swollen or have "water on the knee," and have impaired range of motion. The pain may focus in the knee, but it can radiate out to other parts of the body as well. Typically, your knees will be stiff when you get up in the morning or after a long period of rest, and less so as you move around again, usually improving within twenty minutes. However, the pain may increase the more you use the joint and be alleviated by rest. With advanced osteoarthritis, your knees may hurt even when you aren't using them.

Pain in front of the knee might worsen when you climb stairs, jump, squat, kneel or even sit still for too long (the "theater sign"—

your knees hurt when you stand up at the end of a movie). The knee joint may click, or feel or sound crinkly, crackly or grating (which your doctor will call "crepitus"), especially when you bend the knee as far as it will go and when someone moves your knee for you (as a doctor will in an exam). Knee pain may increase with damp, cool or rainy weather, most likely due to changes in air pressure affecting the fluid within the knee. As OA progresses, your knees may no longer fully bend or extend and can feel unstable—they may buckle, give out, lock or catch—and can even make you limp or fall or become bowlegged.

Arthritis is the most common cause of disability in America and the second most common chronic condition. It causes more limits on daily activity in more people than any other disease. Roughly one in eight Americans has arthritis, and the Centers for Disease Control and Prevention thinks that figure is climbing fast enough to reach almost one fifth of the population (sixty million cases) by 2020. If you look only at people over sixty-five, rates rise to 50 percent. More women than men have arthritis: nearly twenty-seven million women in America, currently. For close to eight million people in this country, arthritis limits everyday activities such as walking, going up stairs, and getting in or out of bed. Roughly six million people believe they have arthritis, but don't have an official diagnosis as such from a doctor— that's 2.5 percent of everyone in the country. Half a million hospitalizations a year are due to arthritis, and estimates of the yearly costs in medical care and economic effects (such as work days missed because of arthritis pain) range from sixty-five to eighty-two *billion* dollars.

PATELLOFEMORAL SYNDROME

Sometimes referred to as "runner's knee," this is the most common cause of pain in the front of the knee, and one of the most common musculoskeletal complaints of any kind in adults. It is really a descriptive term rather than a specific condition—that is, although officially patellofemoral syndrome is a *cause* of knee pain, what it really *is* is knee pain (without changes in cartilage, distinguishing it from arthritis). Patellofemoral syndrome probably involves twenty or thirty—perhaps even as many as one hundred—different specific problems lumped together for the convenience of labeling. There's nothing wrong with that per se, but you should keep in mind that since this condition is no one particular thing, it isn't always heralded by any one symptom or even group of symptoms. Nor will it be solved by any one protocol.

It can start with trauma, overuse, tendinitis, bursitis, dislocation, disease, poor alignment or awkward movement of the parts of the knee. The pain is generally worse after sitting for extended periods of time or after any kind of activity—especially going up stairs or hills, jumping, running or squatting—and usually improves with rest and ice. Typically, a patient has a long history of dull knee pain, with bursts of sharp pain. You will be predisposed to patellofemoral syndrome if you have inflexible leg muscles, malalignment of your kneecaps, undesirable angles within the knee, or poor body alignment or posture. If they are imbalanced, your muscles can actually pull the kneecap too high or too much to one side, interfering with the stability of the joint. Fortunately, this kind of tracking problem is one of the easiest types of knee

29

pain to treat because the right exercises usually correct the problem. (See exercise chapters.)

KNEE INJURIES

All it takes is one blow to the knee or one sudden movement that pushes your knee beyond its normal range of motion and—voilà!—you've entered the wonderful world of knee injury. Most of the time, a knee injury is a strain or torn ligament or tendon, causing pain and swelling in the knee, with the resultant muscle spasm, weakness and difficulty walking. When the tendons can't stretch as much as the force applied demands, you get a tear—a strain or a sprain, depending on the size of the tear. The tear can be anywhere from microscopic ("grade 1") to complete ("grade 4"). Most knee injuries result from twisting the knee, landing a jump, or stopping running abruptly—"noncontact" injuries. The injuries can be acute (one bad jump leaves you sidelined for the season) or the result of overuse (painful knees after years of jump shots). Pain then inhibits your muscles, quickly causing up to a 40 to 60 percent loss of strength, and this sets you up for the potential for further injury.

More than three million Americans injure their knees each year, with about nine hundred thousand of those injuries occurring to the cartilage. The number of women in those ranks is steadily increasing, most likely because of increased participation in sports. This section looks specifically at the most common injuries. Besides direct injuries to the knee covered below, bone fractures of the thigh or shin can create bony fragments that injure other structures in the knee. Infection and tumors or other abnormal growths can also cause knee pain.

Cruciate ligament injury

Injuries to the cruciate ligaments are sometimes called sprains or tears. The ligaments can't stretch as much as the force being applied demands, so they tear, with the damage ranging from microscopic frays to full-thickness tears. The injury may not actually cause pain (then again, it might). Sometimes you just hear a popping sound, and then your leg buckles when you try to take weight on it thanks to a no longer stable knee.

Torn ACLs are the injury of this type you hear the most about, as it seems they are something of an epidemic these days: There are about eighty thousand ACL tears a year in the U.S. And from the looks on the faces of athletes brought down by them, you can tell they cause pretty severe pain. ACLs are usually torn or overstretched by a sudden twisting motion—upper or lower legs go one way, knees the other. PCL injuries usually involve direct impact, as in a car accident or a rugby pileup.

Women are between two and eight times more likely to tear their ACLs than are men involved in comparable activities. This is a classic injury in sports that involve jumping, pivoting and rapid changes in direction, making it very common in those who play basketball, soccer, volleyball and tennis, as well as in skiers. When men injure their ACLs, it almost always involves contact with another player, but for women it rarely does. Seventy percent of reported ACL injuries are noncontact. Not that you have to be an athlete to sustain a torn ACL. Unfortunately, in some cases it occurs when a person is not doing much more than walking down the street and happens to stumble. In fact, chronic structural problems, such as pigeon toes, ankles turning in or out, scoliosis, knock-knees or poor posture, and the repetitive (tiny) traumas they create, are the main causes of this type of injury. The long-term strain and wear and tear set the stage, then one particular jump or turn is the last straw, and your knee goes. If it hadn't happened that way, it would probably have happened another three months down the line when you did something much less dramatic, like roll over in bed.

Collateral ligament injury

The MCL is more often injured than the LCL, usually as the result of a blow to the outside of the knee that stretches or tears the ligament on the inner side. When this happens, you may feel a pop and the knee may buckle to the side. Then comes the pain, swelling and loss of side-to-side stability.

Meniscus injuries

Women are also at greater risk for tearing or damaging these discs of cartilage than are men. The truth is, though, that anyone who exercises regularly has torn or frayed menisci. The meniscus is relatively easy to injure, and it usually happens when you rotate the knee while it is supporting weight. Turning your upper leg while your foot stays planted—twisting to return a serve in a tennis game, for example—is one good way to tear your meniscus. But you can also damage the menisci just by overuse, including simply putting a lot of miles on them, especially when structural issues such as poor posture, leg-length variations or even wide hips, among many other things, put abnormal forces on them. Meniscal damage not related to trauma increases with age. That is, live long enough, exercise long enough, eat poorly enough, or let your strength develop asymmetrically enough, and you'll have meniscal tears.

Usually, chronic meniscal frays don't hurt. When one does hurt, you'll feel it especially when your knee is straightened, though it may well be mild enough not to really interfere with whatever you are doing. Your knee may click or lock, or may just seem weak. Sometimes symptoms clear up without any treatment, and sometimes an old, untreated injury requires treatment only when it flares up months or years later.

Tearing a meniscus acutely—for example, in a skiing accident or the twisting tennis volley described above—is another story. You could have severe pain, especially if the meniscus catches between the bones. You'll get swelling—more or less immediately upon injury or up to several hours later.

Patellar dislocation

This abnormal movement of the kneecap can happen either because of trauma or because of strength imbalance in the quads and hamstrings. Usually, the imbalance exists, and depending on the degree of inequity, a trauma large or small will be the direct trigger. When the kneecap is

What's Worse Than Any One of These?

Two or more of them at the same time! Multiple ligament and/or cartilage strains are the worst. A combination can cause instability of the knee in more than one direction. The knee sort of wobbles with every step, and the shock absorbers are missing. This setup makes further injury and progression to OA a much greater and quicker reality.

pulled out of place, it can get stuck there. The signs of dislocation are pain, usually intense, and a lump on one side of the knee.

Tendinitis and ruptured tendons

Tendinitis, or inflammation of a tendon, is simply the mild end of a scale in which the other end marks a complete tear of the tendon. Either one is most often the result of overuse from activities such as jogging or biking in which the tendon gets worn out, loses much of its elasticity, and gets inflamed as the body tries to repair the damage. You can also get it from sudden movement—such as trying to break a fall—that causes too harsh a contraction—of the quadriceps, for example, though it could be any muscle—tearing the tendons above or below the kneecap. You can also damage the tendons moving from the contracted position toward the relaxed position. If you've ever heard of "jumper's knee," which afflicts many athletes who jump a lot—think basketball and volleyball players— that's a form of tendinitis caused by the strain over time of all those sudden muscle contractions combined with the force of hitting the ground afterward. Older people tend to have weaker tendons, so are more susceptible to injury.

If you have tendinitis, you may feel pain when you are moving fast—for example, running or walking quickly, or jumping. You may have pain or tenderness where the patellar tendon meets the bone, or anywhere along its length. Rupturing a tendon in your knee is very painful. If you completely rupture it, and the muscle is simply no longer connected to the bone, you won't be able to extend or flex the leg. You won't be able to lift your leg up or straighten your knee. If, on the other hand, it is only partially torn or frayed, every movement hurts; either end of the tendon that moves will cause pain.

Iliotibial Band Syndrome

Typical in runners, bikers and dancers, and anyone doing sports that involve forceful landings from jumps or strides, this may be what you're suffering with if you have aching or burning on the side of your thigh toward the knee, which begins not long into running or jumping. The pain may radiate up the side of the thigh. You may feel a pop or a snap when the knee is bent and then straightened, but there usually isn't any swelling and no loss of range of motion. Iliotibial band syndrome is caused by a tendon rubbing over the outer bone of the knee. An injury may be the root cause, but chronic overuse is more likely.

This is one reason running stairs is not usually a good idea for getting in shape. Better you get in shape first and then run stairs—but even then it is very stressful. This was brought home to me when I went hiking in Zion with my brother and sister-in-law. We were changing altitude rather quickly, climbing a lot of switchbacks over steep terrain at a very high angle of incline. But it was coming down that was the killer. We are all generally active people, but our quads were aching by the time we got back to the bottom, and our kneecaps were hurting like crazy from the descent. We all finished the trail walking backward to take some of the strain off. What we should have done was to prepare for this kind of hike by walking up—and especially down—hills in the preceding weeks, just to engage those muscles and get the brain "talking" to the quads, ready for more intense work.

Chondromalacia Patella

This is another wastebasket term for many problems, including deterioration or thinning of the fat pad, cracks of cartilage on the bone, debris from tendinitis, adhesions from bursitis, and more. Whatever the specific source, this softened cartilage on the underside of the kneecap is most commonly injured in young adults, and may result from injury, overuse, misalignment or muscle weakness.

Its trademark is dull pain around or under the kneecap, which is worse when going down stairs or hills. Going up might also be painful, along with any other occasions when the knee has to take weight as it straightens. The knee may sound like sandpaper rubbing as you bend or straighten. It is common among joggers, skiers, bikers and soccer players, and can be aggravated or caused by kneeling. That's why carpet layers and gardeners wear knee pads to protect themselves. The greater protection would be to have healthy cartilage, with no cracks, as you can with the program in this book.

The cartilage is generally damaged by the kneecap rubbing against the thigh bone instead of moving smoothly across it. It can occur following injury that breaks off a piece of cartilage or even bone. Far and away the most common cause is asymmetrical thigh muscle strength resulting in abnormal tracking of the kneecap over the leg bones.

Osteochondritis dissecans

This is caused by the degeneration of the bone under a joint surface due to a lack of blood supply. The problem could be in the bone or on the surface. The bone and the surrounding cartilage loosen and cause pain. It can heal on its own but if it doesn't, cartilage eventually breaks off into the joint, which can cause sharp pain, weakness and locking of the joint. Generally the result of overuse, the condition usually starts with a trauma to the knee, which creates some abnormality in or on the bone.

It can be inherited, though most often it occurs spontaneously in an active young adult, because of either a blockage of a small artery or an unrecognized injury or fracture. This condition is often a precursor to osteoarthritis.

Women's Knees

Women are far more prone to knee pain of all kinds than are men, as you've already seen from some of the facts and figures in this chapter. Add to them: Women are more likely than men to develop chronic pain after trauma, and women are at greater risk of being disabled by their pain. Women's knee pain tends to be cumulative and chronic, while men's usually begins with a specific incident. There's no one definitive explanation for the discrepancy in types and rates of injury and pain as of yet, but theories abound. In the end I'm sure it'll be shown to be a combination of many or all of the ideas currently afloat, so it's worthwhile to be aware of all the leading contenders:

Anatomy

Thanks to a wider pelvis, more flexible hips, and thighs that angle inward from hip to knee more sharply than men's, women's knee ligaments are under a lot more stress than men's. The inside of the knee, in particular, bears a lot of pressure. A wider pelvis also makes the knees angle inward on landing a jump, which can strain the menisci and ligaments, and the knees flex toward each other when changing direction, which can hurt the ACL in particular. Women's knees tend to move inward slightly as they bend, especially in turns or single-leg jumps, with a side to side movement as if the knee were a ball-and-socket rather than a hinge joint. It's a bit of a "knock-kneed" look, and it wreaks havoc on patellar tracking as well as the supporting soft tissues.

Women have looser joints than men. They also have less muscle mass in their thighs in proportion to their body weight. As a result, women have to use their ligaments more to stabilize their knees, whereas men rely more on their muscles to do the job. That means more strain for the ligaments. And since women are, on average, smaller than men, their ligaments, too, are smaller in general, and perhaps therefore more vulnerable.

The dents made by the knobs at the lower end of the thigh bone—known as the "intercondylar notch," through which the all-important ACL ligament must pass—is smaller, on average, in women than in men. The smaller the notch, the smaller—and perhaps weaker—the ligament it can accommodate, and the more friction and wear and tear of the ligament may result.

Women's thigh bones tend to move more forward when they land a jump or crouch, which gives their knees bigger loads to carry. Their shins rotate more, and they are more likely to have their ankles roll inward, both of which have been linked to greater stress on the ACL, raising the risk of injury.

Hormones

Hormones travel in the bloodstream, doing their work all over the body. Hormones work together in complex relationships, so teasing out the effects of just one is never an easy task. One hormone never truly acts all on its own, and it never does just one specific thing, either. While research to date has reached conflicting conclusions about the specifics of how and when and why hormones affect the joints in general and the knee in particular, two things are clear: (1) women face different issues when it comes to their knees than men do, thanks in part to the difference in hormones; and (2) when hormones fall out of balance in women's bodies, the joints will be one of the common places they will notice it.

Chapter Four explores more about hormones and knee injuries.

Physiology

Women's inner ears, which control balance, are wired somewhat differently than men's, and may prove to influence how their bodies move in response to certain stimuli, perhaps in ways that leave them more open to knee injury.

Neuromuscular patterns

Neuromuscular patterns, the interactions between the brain and muscles that dictate how your muscles move and which muscles act when, in what sequence, and how quickly, show gender differences. (Ever been told you "run like a girl"?) Since these patterns are developed rather than inborn, counterproductive ones can be changed through physical conditioning.

Musculature

Women tend to rely more on the muscles in the front of the thigh than those in the back. They have more strength in the front (the quadriceps muscle) than in the back (the hamstrings), whereas in men the relative strengths are more closely balanced. Muscle imbalance alone can lead to injury. Furthermore, when landing a jump, women use the quads more for cushioning, while men rely more on the hamstrings, which turns out to be safer as far as knee injuries go. (Men use the hamstrings three times as much as women do.) Quads tighten the ACL, for example, while the hamstrings take some of the stress off of it. To the degree these differences result from physical training, we can equalize them, which is part of the goal of Chapter Ten.

Biomechanics

Body alignment plays a major role in knee health—and knee injury. Improper alignment, especially appearing "bowlegged" or "knock-kneed," is associated with increased risk of knee injury. The trick here is that your alignment can be off enough to cause you knee problems without you even being aware of it. Fortunately, there are ways you can correct even subtleties to protect your knees, as you'll see in Chapter Three.

Stance

Female athletes tend to stand more upright as they play, whereas men use a more flex-kneed stance. As a result, women tend to hyperextend their knees when moving quickly, which can snap a ligament. Jumping is a particular problem. Men "crouch" approximately twice as much as women.

Shoes

Let's just say the unnatural distribution of weight caused by high heels is no good for the knee. Any heel of two or more inches forces the knee to be and stay flexed (bent) when you walk.

Medical care

Women respond differently than men to many types of treatments, yet most studies focus on men. So women don't always get care tailored to what's best for their bodies. Furthermore, there is some evidence that even well-intentioned doctors respond to women's complaints differently than they do men's, tending toward different explanations for vague complaints and even different treatments, as well as being more likely to dismiss symptoms, thereby letting a condition go untreated.

In the next chapter we'll look more at what contemporary mainstream medicine has to offer for knee pain before focusing on the holistic approaches to women's knees in the remaining chapters.

2

What Mainstream Medicine Has to Offer

Mainstream medicine has a lot to offer for many instances of knee pain. We've got a lot of powerful drugs at our disposal, and if you have an acute trauma, the hospital is definitely the place to be. When surgery and pharmacy are what you really need, modern medicine might as well be the eighth wonder of the world.

The thing is, they aren't always what you need. What mainstream medicine too often lacks is a holistic view of the human body. With expensive or elaborate diagnostic tests, high-tech treatments and dramatic surgeries, very specific knee problems can often be diagnosed and repaired. But more chronic, more amorphous and definitely more common pain usually requires something else for true healing. Often the best mainstream medicine has to offer in these cases is symptom management, which isn't always satisfactory and often comes with unpleasant or even dangerous side effects. Even the most slam-dunk mainstream techniques sometimes simply don't work. Or, they work in as much as the ligament is now back more or less where it started out, for instance, but nagging pain and the cause of the problem still remain. And if the true cause of the problems are not addressed, the problem progresses and symptoms can return again and again when the acute therapies are stopped.

Contemporary medicine also has a tendency to brush off complaints it can't clearly explain the cause of—with a particular bad track record when it comes to women. I'm here to tell you there is help to be had, even if you've been told there's "nothing wrong"—or nothing to be done about it.

Underneath it all is the fact that modern medicine generally focuses on disease, but not on why we get disease in the first place, and, therefore, how to *not* get disease. With about one trillion dollars spent each year for health care in this country, less than 1 percent goes toward prevention efforts. Though this is changing, as more people seek complementary preventions and remedies, the money by and large isn't going to crucial root causes, either. So we too often fail to maintain a clean environment or eliminate toxins or address other underlying causes of much disease, and we pay for the consequences with our most precious commodity—our health.

This chapter looks at how to make use of all the best mainstream medicine has to offer. But we'll also expand our scope to point out additional, and too often overlooked, paths to healing that many women with knee pain need—instead of or in addition to mainstream approaches—all of which will be explored in greater depth in coming chapters.

Doctors

Your first stop will probably be your regular general doctor, who should certainly be your ally and advocate. But it is important to determine if he or she really knows about knees or not. Do not settle for a shrugging off of your problem, or a simple statement that there's nothing to be done. The sooner you take action, the better your chances of preventing a small problem from becoming a big one—and of getting rid of it altogether. So seek help from the appropriate physician or specialist when necessary.

Physiatrists, sports medicine specialists, and *osteopaths* should all be well versed in knees, and will be the most likely to have at least exercises, if not nutritional approaches, to suggest. You might also be referred to a *physical therapist* (PT). *Orthopedic surgeons* are who many people with knee diseases or knee injuries go to; "orthopods" should be trained, well versed, and open to nonsurgical as well as surgical treatment of bones and joints and the surrounding ligaments, tendons and muscles. For arthritis in the knee, a *rheumatologist*, specializing in arthritis, may be your choice.

The fact of the matter is, however, that most specialists, surgical or not, deal with repairing a problem that already exists. This book can help you do that, but better still, you'll learn here how to prevent problems and reverse the cause of your symptoms before serious damage is done. More than treating disease, the information in this book will help you normalize function—in the knee itself, in the entire body, and at the cellular level.

Whichever health-care practitioners you end up seeing, good team work—between them, as well as between you and them—is invaluable. For example, I never simply write out a prescription for physical therapy; I like to call the therapist directly to share my impressions and ask for his or her input. Make sure your caregivers are willing to communicate with each other, and with you. You should always drive the decision-making machine in relation to your health care.

Tools for Diagnoses

I do a thorough and careful knee exam on my patients before I design a treatment plan. If that doesn't give a good diagnosis, I may order an X ray or an MRI, or ask for consultation with another doctor. Or I may recommend a trial of therapy, which consists of a program designed to address what I have found and what I already know about her general lifestyle patterns. On new patients, I think a thorough physical and personal history are important prior to treating knee pain of unknown cause.

If you follow the program in this book regarding diet, nutritional supplements and exercise, you should be improving within six weeks. In the cases in which my patients are not considerably better at the six-week mark (or are getting worse before then), I have them get an X ray or an MRI or other more involved tests, looking for a bone spur or other specific problem that I didn't find on my initial evaluation and which needs a more drastic or different kind of intervention. I don't usually use those tests sooner unless the patient is definitely headed for surgery or there is a concern about a serious or unusual problem. In most usual knee problems, unless surgery is a given, the results of those tests probably won't change the treatment program anyway.

Generally speaking, mainstream medicine is quicker with the expensive diagnostic tests. But in any event, the diagnostic process always begins with a history and physical. The doctor will ask you for details about your symptoms (local to your knee as well as systemic, such as chills and fever), any injury you've had, your general health—especially any condition that might be causing pain—and your activities. Be prepared to describe your pain specifically (type, intensity, duration, locations, timing), to state how and when it started, and to be as precise as possible about exactly how any injury occurred (What exactly were you doing? What position was your knee in? Did you hear anything, such as a pop or a tear? What did it feel like? Did anything hit your knee—and how hard and in what direction? Could you get up/take weight on it/walk on your own right afterward?). You should also explain when and how your pain interferes with your usual activities, what makes it better, and what makes it worse.

Your doctor should have many questions for you, and as many relevant details as you can provide will help in getting a good diagnosis. This is the first and most important step to discovering the best treatment approach. Whether or not you are specifically asked, you'll want to mention any previous knee problems; if the pain has gotten better or worse; anything you've noticed that worsens or alleviates the pain; if you feel anything moving inside your knee; if you've had any recent changes in your usual activities (including what shoes you wear and what protective equipment you wear while exercising) or workout routines; what kind of exercise you get and how you warm up for it; and what your knee did and how it looked after an injury.

Your doctor will also manipulate your knee, bending, straightening, rotating and pressing it to feel for injury, test the limits of motion, assess stability and pinpoint the pain. He or she will also watch you sit, stand, walk and perhaps run; test your muscle strength; feel for your pulse and test sensation in your legs and feet. Doctors will be looking for swelling, muscle atrophy, gait, alignment, fluid, masses, locking, joint stability, clicks and much more. They will perform "stress tests" by pushing and pulling your knee in certain directions to see how your body and knee deal with this stress. Each knee, and each leg, should be compared against the other.

Done well and thoroughly, these approaches should be sufficient to diagnose 90 percent of all knee problems. For the remaining 10 percent, there are several helpful tests available. I'll review the most widely used here.

X RAYS

X rays provide the familiar two-dimensional view of your knee bones. Their usefulness is actually pretty limited when it comes to knee pain, however. The main issue is that cartilage doesn't show in an X ray; nor do ligaments, tendons or menisci. That makes X rays mainly suitable for identifying and visualizing fractures, arthritis, cysts, tumors and degenerative changes. They can also be used to measure kneecap angles to understand how the kneecap tracks (although they are too infrequently used for this purpose, considering how important that information can be). X rays are sometimes necessary to confirm a diagnosis, especially for insurance claims such as workers' compensation. Beyond that, X rays can reveal alignment problems, dislocation and arthritis that has progressed so far as to create bone damage and loss of joint space (when so much cartilage has been lost that the bones move closer together), though those things can usually be diagnosed by thorough history and physical.

X rays are dramatically overused. One study revealed that just 7 percent of X rays in adults with knee pain showed fractures—not surprising, since about three-quarters of the patients X rayed had no reason to suspect they had a fracture. Researchers estimated that at least half of the patients could—and should—have done without the wasted expense and exposure of the X ray.

Many of those unnecessary X rays were most likely done on patients with knee pain from arthritis or other chronic problems. Because painful cartilage damage precedes the bone damage X rays can reveal, and cartilage doesn't show up on an X ray, this can be the path to hearing "there's nothing wrong" from your doctor. There is most definitely something wrong (your knee pain is telling you)—it's just that your doctor can't see it! And even if your doctor does see something, realize that there is no direct correspondence between the degree of pain and stiffness experienced and the extent of damage seen in X rays. The same bony changes were there last week when you had *no* knee pain.

I don't routinely X ray anyone initially, except patients with significant problems with no apparent cause or when there are systemic symptoms such as infections or toxicity. I do use X rays on occasions when I want to watch the progression of arthritis without doing a series of MRIs.

CT Scans (CAT scans)
(Computerized Axial Tomography)

CT scans combine a series of cross-section images—each one a "slice" of the knee—to provide a three-dimensional view. CT scans can show soft tissue (tendons, ligaments, muscle and cartilage) somewhat more clearly than regular X rays, but are best used to see bone in the clearest detail. You can see all the layer and depth of the bone, which cannot be seen on an X ray. CT scan technology removes the shadowing effects of skin, muscle, fat, fluid, etc., thereby improving the visualization of the bone dramatically over a regular X ray. CT scans are used mostly to find fractures. I can't remember ever ordering a CT of the knee; I use mostly X ray and MRI (see below) instead. The fact of the matter is that an MRI will show most anything about the knee that a CT scan might, and without the X ray exposure.

MRI (Magnetic Resonance Imaging)

MRIs also combine cross-sections for a three-dimensional view, usually of specific parts of the knee, and are called for when you are looking for soft tissue. But MRI is not an X ray—there is no radiation exposure. Instead, magnetic fields are used to create an image. (This is why you can't use an MRI if you have a metal implant anywhere in your body— the magnetic field is too strong and will pull the metal to it.) MRI is good for pinpointing damage or disease of ligaments, tendons, muscles and cartilage, as well as bleeding, infection, tumors and inflammation.

Most injuries don't require it, however; a good exam and history will usually suffice. I use MRI when something about the physical exam doesn't make sense, when the severity of the injury makes it impossible to do a thorough exam, or when I think surgery is immediately required (without an attempt at more conservative treatment first).

MRI is most often employed by orthopedic surgeons to guide surgery, deal with extensive ligament damage, confirm a diagnosis, or provide documentation for insurance purposes. MRIs get less accurate the older you get because all tissues deteriorate over time (i.e., as you get older). The deterioration shows on an MRI, with no way to differentiate whether or not the cause is anything other than benign, or if it is causing you any symptoms. An MRI shows all tissue, normal and abnormal, but there is no way to know which if any of it has bearing on your immediate problem. For the same reason, MRIs must be interpreted differently in patients who have had previous knee surgery or who have arthritis so far gone it will show up on a regular, old-fashioned X ray.

The biggest drawback of MRI is that it tells you only what is anatomically abnormal, not why you have pain. To give you an example from my personal experience, I recently had an MRI of my wrist after an injury. Based on the results, the doctor recommended surgery—on a problem on the side of my wrist opposite from where I was having pain. The MRI showed some abnormal tissue that was causing no symptoms. Unfortunately, it didn't reveal anything about what *was* bothering me. (I declined the surgery, thank you very much.)

Just because a better technology exists doesn't mean it always needs to be used. For example: Nearly 90 percent of meniscal tears will be picked up via MRI—the same percentage that can be correctly diagnosed by a good physical exam alone. Most doctors agree that MRIs miss at least 20 percent of pathologies—and some say it is more like 80 percent. In my opinion, about half the time, an MRI provides information not pertinent to the patient's condition. MRIs can miss things that are there, and can show things that *are* there but have nothing to do with the problem the patient is experiencing. It is always amazing to see what is found on an arthroscopic exam (see below) that wasn't found on the MRI.

Bone Scans (Radionucleotide Scanning)

Bone scans detect blood flow to the bone and cell activity within bone. This is good for seeing tumors, degenerative processes, inflammatory processes and discrete fractures.

Arthroscopy (Arthroscopic Surgery)

Arthroscopy is a surgical procedure used to both diagnose and treat knee problems. A tiny camera inserted through small incisions (about as wide as a pencil) gives doctors a direct look at cartilage, tendons and ligaments in the knee joint to assess damage, and guides instruments used to repair them. Because it is invasive, you'd most likely get arthroscopy only if the doctor intends to repair at the same time he or she is diagnosing. There are risks attendant to any surgery, such as infection and anesthesia problems. (More on this later.)

Aspiration

Aspiration—using a needle placed under the kneecap or into the knee to draw off fluid accumulated in the knee—is rarely used for treatment, since it comes with some risk of developing a serious infection and/or early onset arthritis, and fluid may well just build back up again. Fluid removed this way can be tested for signs of infection, gout and some kinds of arthritis, though not the osteoarthritis we mainly discuss in this book. Blood in the fluid indicates a serious injury, such as a fracture or a tear in ligament or cartilage, while a buildup of clear fluid most likely means it is just an old injury or underlying condition that has been irritated or aggravated. Aspiration can also be used to relieve symptoms such as stiffness, pain and swelling, as we'll cover later in this chapter. If you do need it, make sure it is done by an experienced hand.

The right diagnosis is key to getting rid of knee pain now and forever, so neither you nor your doctor should be in any rush to decide exactly what is going on. Don't settle for snap diagnoses, but don't feel the need to push for high-tech tests just because your doctor has access to the machinery, either. Doctors should never treat an X ray or a lab test—they should treat only the patients themselves. If some diagnostic test doesn't jibe with what the patient is telling me, or with what I find on physical exam, I believe the patient and my exam over the testing, and I'll get a consultation from another medical professional if I can't successfully integrate the different forms of information.

While your doctor has to pin a generic label on your condition for the purposes of filing insurance forms, the real diagnosis should be tailored to your particular life, set of symptoms, and circumstances. And, of course, you should never have to live with the conclusion that nothing's wrong, or that nothing can be done about it. If your knees hurt, they hurt—and there are clear and simple approaches to relieving the pain whether or not they are in any given doctor's or insurance company's standard playbook.

Treating Knee Pain

The most important thing to aim for in treating knee pain—or any pain, for that matter—is that treatment should be geared not just to limiting the symptoms but to healing the root cause of the problem. Symptoms are simply the body's announcement that something is out of balance, and treatment should be about restoring that balance. Much of what conventional Western medicine currently has to offer aims only at the symptoms, without addressing the underlying issues. The program in this book is designed to get to the heart of the matter for the majority of cases of knee pain.

In the context of conventional Western medicine, the specific treatment that is right for you depends on the specific diagnosis, of course. Responses to any given approach are highly individual (what worked for your neighbor may not be the right thing for you), and in many cases there aren't good studies proving the efficacy of standard treatments. Besides, how standard are you? Are your body, mind, and spirit the same as those of your neighbors, your friends, or even your sister? As Sir William Osler, one of the nineteenth century's most prominent physicians, said: Doctors should treat people who have diseases—not diseases that have people.

This section, then, is meant to give you a brief rundown of the most likely medical, surgical and therapeutic options you may end up discussing with your doctor, including notable benefits—and drawbacks. As you contemplate your ultimate choices, it is worth keeping in mind that placebos work about 30 percent of the time, and "mind-body" techniques such as meditation and visualization can work up to 80 percent of the time. The rest of this book has a lot of options to offer you. But we'll begin where most people do with their regular doctors: with mainstream medicine's answers. We'll start with the most straight forward and least invasive.

LOSING WEIGHT

Taking off even a few pounds will decrease pressure on the joints. This is a crucial factor in osteoarthritis in particular. And excess weight also stresses support structures such as ligaments, cartilage, muscles, etc. Losing weight will only ease your suffering.

RICE

This is a basic approach for the immediate aftermath of some injuries, meant to assuage pain and swelling: Rest, Ice, Compression, Elevation. Rest, at the time of the injury, prevents additional damage to the injured area. You should resume normal activities as soon as possible, without increasing the damage to the tissue. Ice packs for about ten minutes every two hours are recommended for the first two to three days after an injury to reduce internal bleeding and control swelling and inflammation. You should not use ice for more than twenty minutes at a time; while it decreases inflammation, it also decreases circulation and, with it, the body's ability to bring healing resources to the site and remove debris from it. Compression (as with a gently wrapped elastic bandage) and elevation also increase the amount of blood and lymph flowing from an injured area to combat swelling and inflammation. You might also want to use pain relievers, such as those described later in this chapter.

If the pain is severe or lasts more than a couple days, you should consult your doctor, and if it continues for more than a week and your doctor doesn't have good strategies at hand, consider seeing a knee specialist. Don't ignore an injury, even if it seems relatively minor, as unaddressed damage can set you up for knee and other problems down the road, even if it doesn't slow you down now.

PRICE

This adds "position" to the formula above. It isn't always necessary, but often basic treatment will include the use of a brace of some kind to immobilize and/or stabilize the joint and prevent abnormal motion. For many injuries, this is meant to be only a short-term approach, for no more than a day, to get swelling to go down. Prolonged immobilization will result in muscle weakness and wasting.

MEAT

The latest thinking on treating most knee injuries improves upon RICE, recommending Movement, Exercise, Analgesia and Treatment.

The sooner you get to normal movement patterns, the more quickly and more fully you will recover. The idea is not to disrupt the normal brain-to-muscle pathways. Recovery is faster when you don't have to unlearn newly acquired bad habits such as limping or protecting your knee with other abnormal movements. Athletes in peak condition show deconditioning of their muscles within twenty-four hours of non-use—and it takes up to two days for them to recover to their original level. Keeping moving is no less important for those of us in less than tip-top shape. The lesson is: The quicker you get on top of the situation, the less time you'll need to spend catching up.

SPLINT, BRACE, CAST, ELASTIC BANDAGE OR NEOPRENE SLEEVE

Popular though they are, knee braces have not been proven effective at preventing injuries, and so are not generally recommended. However, they can add stability to an unstable joint, and can be useful when recovering from injuries. Wearing them during everyday activities can prevent further damage while your knee recovers.

HEAT

A few days after an injury, switch to heat rather than ice, to increase the blood supply to the area and promote healing. Try a heating pad or hot pack—local heat is better than a full body bath. Warmth increases the flow of blood, oxygen, nutrients and lymph to the injury and also increases the removal of the debris.

ORTHOTICS

Orthotics are a wonderful tool, but don't give in to the temptation to view them as a cure-all. If your knee and body have alignment problems before you get orthotics, you'll likely still have them afterward—and the orthotics can in fact exaggerate them. You'll get worse, rather than better. You might get lifts because of a diagnosis that one leg is longer than the other, but maybe that appears to be the case because your pelvis isn't level. If one side of the pelvis is higher than the other because of muscle spasm rather than bone length, then one leg will appear to be shorter than the other, and a lift will only exacerbate the problem. First fix your alignment, then use orthotics to compensate for any anatomical imbalances that remain in your feet. Foot and arch orthotics are designed to be used to address foot problems, not knee problems.

EXERCISE

Simple, low-impact exercises can restore joint movement and strengthen the knee. Low-impact functional exercise strengthens muscles without stressing joints. That means exercise done slowly enough to allow your muscles to engage with increasing levels and to allow you to stabilize the joint as the knee absorbs the full weight and force of your body. Stretching and flexibility are important too.

PHYSICAL THERAPY

Physical therapy is designed to ease any pain, alleviate inflammation and swelling, and get your knee in shape so it does everything you ask it to do easily and well—in other words, normalize function and ability. Whether you are dealing with chronic pain or rehabbing after an injury, you will first work on your range of motion before moving on to improving muscle tone and eventually building strength, flexibility and, finally, agility. PT *before* surgery might obviate the need for surgery— and if not, then at least it will set you up to recover as smoothly and quickly as possible. Every surgery should be followed by a course of physical therapy. There are great protocols that speed up healing and recovery. PT not only gets you back in action but also protects you from injuring yourself again, in the same or in a new way.

Physical therapy is meant to get you back to normal functioning. Relieving pain, strengthening muscles, getting rid of excess fluid and all those specifics are only part of the goal. The main thing is to reeducate the body as to what normal and good function should be. Any physical therapy that aims for less is, in my opinion, inadequate.

Exactly how physical therapy accomplishes that goal varies with the individual. Two people with the same knee surgery from the same injury can require totally different courses of PT because they bring to the table different personal qualities, different bodily builds, different musculatures, different abilities to heal, different life experiences. PT that treats every knee with the same protocol will only be successful in a certain percentage of patients. It is only when the physical therapist— like any other kind of medical practitioner—looks at you as an individual, and as a whole person, that you can get the most out of it. You need a program designed just for you. It may involve ultrasound, strengthening machines, phono- or iontophoresis (ways of directing current and heat to more specific levels and areas, treating, for example, only the superficial muscles or only the bone and deep muscles), medication, hot packs, ice and more. But how much, when, in what sequence, and in what ratio? That should be determined for you alone.

More than just strength training for weak muscles, PT should also include training in sequence of muscle firing (the order in which muscles contract determines how normal the function of the knee can be); coordinating different muscles; disinhibiting muscles that have been "turned off" because of pain; and repatterning brain-to-muscle signals that help you sense where your body is in space and how it is moving—all of which are needed to reestablish normal function. You'll be aiming to equalize the strength of muscles that affect both knees, not only for the aesthetics but also for proper alignment and bodily balance.

You must normalize function before you strengthen the muscles. Once that's done, in most cases, PT for sore knees of any stripe will focus on strengthening each of the individual muscles around your knee to provide more support to the knee and stabilize the joint. As an example, you may need to strengthen your medial quad (on the inside of the knee) more than your lateral quad (on the outside of the knee) to normalize the tracking of your kneecap (see Chapter Ten). The end result should be symmetrical strength in appropriate proportions in all the muscles around the joint.

Your physical therapist should advise you on how to modify your activities and techniques to prevent future injury. In addition to guiding you through exercises during your regular appointments and monitoring your progress, he or she should teach you exercises to do at home, all of which should be tailored to the kind of activity you do regularly, as well as to your age, size, fitness level, muscularity and motivation. (Serious athletes may also want to work with an athletic trainer.)

Physical therapists use many techniques other than exercise, including galvanic stimulation (a type of electrical stimulation used to get the muscles working and to reduce pain); ultrasound; micro-current (a form of ultrasound using much lower levels of current, which mimic the body's own electrical current); cold lasers; phonophoresis/iontophoresis; hydrotherapy and more. You won't need all of them, but it is nice if your physical therapist has them available if your physician requests them. Whatever your PT ends up consisting of, you should get not simply the standard PT protocol for your diagnosis but an individualized program designed specifically for you, as a whole person who happens to have a knee problem.

ELECTRICAL STIMULATION

Electrical stimulation directs current to contract specific muscles in order to move fluid, reduce inflammation, stop pain and/or begin muscle training. Whether done in your doctor's or physical therapist's office, or with a small portable unit at home, the main goals are usually to modify the brain's perception of painful stimuli so that the brain helps to send, and the muscle is more ready to accept, normal stimuli, and to strengthen the muscles.

ANALGESICS

Pain relievers such as acetaminophen (Tylenol) and the narcotic codeine provide welcome relief from knee pain for some people, but of course treat only the symptom of pain while doing nothing about inflammation or the underlying problem. Not all pain is associated with inflammation, however, so these are sometimes the correct choice. Like every drug, these come with some risk of side effects, up to and including liver or kidney failure. (Regular acetaminophen users' risk of chronic kidney failure increases up to 2.5 times, depending on total lifetime intake, and there have been reported cases of death due to liver failure from even short-term use.)

Some research indicates analgesics may work less well for women than for men. Some people don't get as much relief as with NSAIDs (see below), but acetaminophen and codeine come with less risk of serious GI side effects. The rate at which patients are choosing to use acetaminophen is increasing; one recent decade-long study showed a doubling, up to 10 percent, in arthritis patients using it, most likely because it seems to be a "safer" choice. (However, this increase in use of these drugs may also mean that the number of people dealing with pain is increasing.)

NSAIDS (NON-STEROIDAL ANTI-INFLAMMATORY DRUGS)

Pain relievers such as aspirin, Aleve, and ibuprofen are already the most commonly recommended and used therapies for knee pain, slightly expanding on "take two aspirin and call me in the morning." New entries into the NSAIDs category called COX-2 inhibitors (including Bextra, Vioxx and Celebrex) have been heavily advertised to consumers as well as doctors since their introduction in 1999.

NSAIDs are really good at relieving pain for a lot of people. However, over time they may, in a roundabout way, speed up progression of osteoarthritis, interfere with cartilage repair mechanisms, and even promote the destruction of cartilage. These medicines also have significant potential for serious toxic side effects, particularly gastrointestinal upset and damage (including ulcers and hemorrhage) and liver and/

or kidney damage. Regular aspirin use increases your risk of kidney failure up to two and a half times, again related to how much you've taken over a lifetime. Sustained use of NSAIDs triples the risk of serious gastrointestinal side effects such as ulcers and bleeding, according to one survey of nearly fifty top-drawer studies (which did not look at COX-2 inhibitors).

NSAIDs are designed to block an enzyme known as cyclooxygenase-2 (COX-2) because it causes inflammation. When COX-2 is blocked, prostaglandin synthesis is inhibited, which results in an anti-inflammatory effect and pain relief. But NSAIDs also interfere with COX-1, which is supposed to serve to protect the GI tract, liver, kidney and platelets that help your blood clot. Newer NSAIDs—selective COX-2 inhibitors (Celebrex, Vioxx, Bextra)—leave COX-1 alone to do its duty, and so appear somewhat safer, though we don't yet know much about their long-term effects. However, COX-2 inhibitors have been linked to heart problems, high blood pressure, kidney damage and failure, and even meningitis (inflammation of membranes surrounding the brain and spinal cord), and have been shown to retard healing of fractures, at least in lab animals. People taking Vioxx have a quadrupled risk of heart attack compared to those on aspirin or ibuprofen.

NSAIDs side effects are more common and more serious in older patients. Research shows that virtually everyone over fifty who takes NSAIDs for three months or more will have some degree of stomach ulcers (microscopic though they may be—at least at first). Over sixteen thousand people being treated for arthritis in the U.S. die each year of GI bleeding caused by NSAIDs.

It's no wonder arthritis patients' NSAIDs use has been declining over the last ten years or so. Still, these drugs are prescribed more than

80 million times a year in the U.S. alone, accounting for 4.5 percent of all prescriptions—and that doesn't take into account the surely even more common over-the-counter versions. COX-2 inhibitors, such as Celebrex, Vioxx, and Bextra, are the best-selling arthritis drugs. In 2001, Celebrex was the tenth best-selling drug in the country (with 24.5 million prescriptions), and Vioxx thirteenth (23.7 million prescriptions). That's a multibillion dollar business for their makers.

As with analgesics, NSAIDs do nothing to slow or stop the mechanical problem that is causing the pain, and can't protect against joint damage. They do what their full name says they do: fight inflammation and the attendant pain.

Despite studies galore, each asserting an edge of one drug over another in some narrowly defined parameter, there are no definitive conclusions as to which NSAID (if any) is superior. In fact, a recent study analyzing results of eighty of the best drug trials done to date showed little difference in effectiveness among them, and negative side effects in all of them. It isn't even clear that the expensive prescriptions offer any more benefits than the pills readily available in your grocery or drug store. What works best for you will be very individual, in terms of relieving your pain and avoiding side effects. A study by an insurance organization (obviously, a vested interest) found that the vast majority of people taking fancier prescription drugs in a bid to avoid GI side effects weren't actually at any risk of those side effects from the older, cheaper, more readily available drugs in the first place—and about half took enough aspirin, intending to protect their hearts, to counteract any GI edge the newer drugs had anyway. The insurance companies surely don't want to pay more for what may be no safer or more effective, and neither should you, especially when we know much less about their long-term effects than we do about older drugs.

My advice is to be wary of overblown advertising claims, weigh your risk of side effects carefully, and be mindful of the high costs for prescription drugs that may or may not be any more helpful to you—and be sure to have your doctor follow you closely in case any negative effects do crop up. Your doctors should probably start you off with an over-the-counter remedy, moving on to a generic prescription such as naproxen if necessary, before casting your lot in with the flashy newer products.

My *best* advice, however, is that if you need anti-inflammatories or pain relief, try the safer natural remedies first (see Chapter Nine).

TOPICAL ANESTHETICS

There are topical liquids, creams or gels, including but not limited to NSAIDs, aspirin, herbs, homeopathics, and hot pepper creams such as capsaicin and others. They are safe because they are not systemic and don't involve the liver or kidneys. They can be anti-inflammatory and can deplete your substance P. Substance P is found in the nerve endings and it must be present for you to perceive pain. Depleting it will reduce the sensation of pain.

Topical NSAIDs can be just as effective as their oral counterparts, and they are always safer. Studies have shown that using a topical hot pepper cream can as much as double the effectiveness of oral NSAIDs.

ANTIDEPRESSANTS

Medications such as Paxil, Zoloft, Celexa and Elavil (in fact, probably all antidepressants) can be used in chronic pain situations to reset the brain's thermostat for the perception of pain, changing the pain threshold so your level of pain sensitivity decreases.

I'm not talking about knee pain as a depressive issue. You might be depressed because you are in pain, and antidepressants might help out there, but I want to be clear that you are not feeling pain only because you are depressed.

STEROID INJECTIONS

Corticosteroids may relieve pain temporarily, but unless your problem is totally inflammatory, they won't change the root cause of the pain. Few studies exist proving the usefulness of corticosteroids this way, and when they do work, the effect is short-lived (perhaps a few weeks). However, for acute episodes of pain, it is an inexpensive and relatively safe option. But you still must be careful: Injecting into a tendon can also increase your risk of rupturing that tendon; overuse in a joint can actually weaken cartilage and promote arthritis. So the general recommendation is no more than three shots in any given year in any given joint. The shot itself can cause pain, so you might want to ice the site repeatedly for a day or two afterward.

HYALURONATE INJECTIONS

Hyaluronate is a fluid found naturally in healthy knee cartilage, serving to lubricate and cushion the knee joint. Knee osteoarthritis may decrease or debase this fluid. The injected version is supposed to supplement or replace what your body makes, helping decrease pain linked to cartilage damage and improve mobility and function. Some studies show it does so more effectively than oral placebo medicines and even NSAIDs (naproxen) for osteoarthritis, with fewer side effects. In fairness I must note that other studies comparing hyaluronate injections to placebo injections yielded similar results for each. Still, some work indicates that about three-quarters of patients report feeling better with hyaluronate than with anything else they've tried, with benefits lasting months to years. Many people experience complete relief with these injections, even for vigorous activity such as running or tennis. These injections work well enough to get some patients off the track to knee replacement surgery—or at least delay such drastic interventions, eliminating pain while waiting for them.

It is important to note, however, that the best results seem to come in the least advanced cases—the ones most likely to respond to a totally noninvasive program such as the one in this book. For this reason, I never do these injections. They work well if you have minor damage, but so do the supplements and herbal remedies described here, with fewer potential side effects. And the injections work poorly in more serious cases—and frequently don't prevent the need for surgery.

For those who do pursue this course, more studies are still needed to amass good evidence about how to best use this technique, including dosing, the type of hyaluronate, and how often you can repeat the treatment. The usual course of treatment currently involves a series of three injections a couple of weeks apart, with no particular promises about how long any beneficial effects will last.

Be forewarned: Many insurance policies don't currently cover hyaluronate injections.

ASPIRATION

Fluid built up in the knee is sometimes removed with a well placed needle to relieve pain, although it's mainly fallen out of favor, since ice and NSAIDs or analgesics should be enough to do the trick. The most common uses of this practice are probably after dislocation and for diagnostic purposes (to see what is in the fluid).

SURGERY

Surgical techniques have improved dramatically and continue to improve. Knee surgeries are becoming less invasive and more specific, and therefore less traumatic than they once were, allowing more manageable recoveries. Still, with the exception of athletes who need to resume playing as quickly as possible, surgery is usually the treatment of last resort—as it should be.

Surgery is usually effective when it is truly indicated, but all surgery has risks associated with it, so you don't want to undertake it lightly. Not least in this situation is that any knee surgery can lead to chronic knee problems. Even so, there are over two million knee surgeries each year in the U.S., mostly to menisci and ligaments—not counting procedures on the bones themselves. Data from 1995 shows three types of knee surgery combined to make up fully 5 percent of all outpatient surgeries. It pays to remember, too, that sometimes even surgery doesn't (or can't) fix your pain.

For most people, the program in this book should be able to help you avoid surgery. More than three-quarters of cases of patellofemoral syndrome, to take just one example, will improve without surgery, and surgery should be used only if several months of physical therapy, limitations of aggravating movements and activities, and other healing techniques mentioned later in this book don't provide satisfactory results. There are some acute problems for which surgery is indicated sooner rather than later. These include things such as bad skiing or other athletic injuries in which multiple serious damages have occurred. But most often, what you need is patience; no one should leap immediately to surgery for chronic knee pain.

There are many types of surgery, so you really can't generalize about how long it takes to recover from surgery, what to expect from the recovery period, or if you can expect to be 100 percent after surgery. Surgeons who handle the tissue with gentleness and in a respectful manner do the least damage to the tissue, so the body has less trauma to repair and heal from. Surgeons who look at you as a whole person instead of "a knee" are always my preference.

If you do need surgery, this program is still of great value, and will help you go into surgery in the best possible shape and make the course of recovery as smooth as possible—and protect against reinjury or other relapse.

We'll take a look at the most common types of surgery here.

Arthroscopy

Camera-guided surgery through tiny incisions, as described earlier, is useful for treatment as well as for diagnosis. Surgeons use many different specific approaches—including but not limited to cartilage grafting, removal of bone or scar tissue, shaving down bone spurs, and taking out loose tissue fragments—many of which can be grouped into two basic techniques: lavage (using saline to rinse physical and chemical irritants out of the joint) and debridement (trimming or scraping rough cartilage or ligaments). It's quick (as far as surgery goes) and usually done without requiring a hospital stay. It costs about five thousand dollars.

About 400,000 to 650,00 people go under the knife this way each year in the U.S. A sizeable majority of those patients head to the OR because of arthritis, but new research shows that *arthroscopy is almost completely ineffective for arthritis.* In a rarely seen approach, an orthopedic surgeon at a Texas veteran's hospital compared arthroscopy and a placebo: actually, fake surgery. The real procedure yielded no better results than the sham. The results were impressive enough to make the surgeon declare he'd no longer perform arthroscopy (as well as for the *New England Journal of Medicine* to publish them). Arthroscopy is also frequently performed on patients with patellofemoral pain, yet less than half benefit from it.

Arthroscopic surgery *is* good for some conditions, particularly torn ligaments or menisci. Torn ligaments are frequently replaced—with ligaments cut from elsewhere in your body, or from a cadaver—rather than repaired. If you experience pain that starts intensely and all at once, or knees that "catch," lock or give way, thanks to loose meniscus or cartilage, you could benefit from arthroscopy. Even patients with arthritis (though usually less so in an advanced case) could benefit, if they have some of those same mechanical symptoms. Rough surfaces can be smoothed, bone spurs can be trimmed, debris can be removed from joints, and in some cases cartilage can be repaired or replaced. But pain alone should not be enough to indicate surgery.

Arthroscopy can't, of course, address many of the issues underlying knee pain, such as excess weight, weak muscles, an unstable joint or poor alignment. And it may very well remove signs of damage to the joint, such as frayed or torn menisci or bone spurs, without relieving the symptoms. Knee pain that is the result of other things, such as poor mechanics, emotions, and misuse, won't be relieved.

In any event, you should try all the less invasive approaches previously mentioned before resorting to surgery. Be prepared: These other nonsurgical options can take six to twelve weeks to prove effective, and could take as long as a year. But be patient. In my opinion, it is more prudent to take the time to see if your pain can be corrected or managed in another way before rushing into surgery and all the risks associated with it.

Pam

Pam, an active woman in her early sixties, had arthroscopic surgery on her knees—twice!—because she had pain when she exercised. Both times (two years apart) she went diligently to physical therapy both before and after the surgery, but both times the pain returned when she went back to her usual hour a day on the treadmill. She'd had her torn meniscus repaired, her chondromalacia addressed, and various pieces of debris removed from her knees, all to no avail. Images taken after the second surgery showed loss of cartilage in the middle of the knee, and early arthritic spur formation. Pam thought her fate was sealed—and it didn't look like it would include the active lifestyle she was accustomed to, at least not without nagging pain.

Out of options (or so she thought), Pam was finally ready to try what I'd suggested to her at the outset: eating to heal her knees. Insulin resistant and overweight despite her good aerobic-exercise habits, Pam started somewhat half-heartedly on a diet program like the one described in Chapter Five. Before long she noticed some improvement in her knees, and thereupon became a die-hard convert. She started going for weekly coaching sessions with a well-known nutritionist, and fully committed to following the plan quite intensely. She also began working with a personal trainer three times a week, and going to the gym twice a week on her own, switching a good bit of her time from aerobics to weight training. Three months into changing the way she ate, Pam was able to work out with no pain for the first time in years. What the best surgical techniques couldn't do for her body, Pam did for herself.

Reconstructive surgery

Reconstructive surgery includes a variety of procedures addressing a range of symptoms and conditions. It is "open" surgery, as opposed to the small incisions of arthroscopy, and includes procedures such as total knee replacement, though that gets its very own section, coming up next. Surgeons can reattach ruptured tendons; fix cartilage; put bone fragments back in place or remove them in such a way as to increase the blood supply to the area; remove small pieces of bone that should not be there; put in hardware such as screws, wires and plates; and much more—using too many techniques to detail here.

This is not a simple repair. It involves reconstructing (as the name suggests) the many moveable, bony parts and some or all of the soft tissues that attach to them and/or hold them together. Reconstructive surgery can be partial or total, addressing problems ranging from something needing a minor repair to total destruction of the knee caused by a severe skiing injury.

Osteochondral autograft transplantation

Osteochondral autograft transplantation—which, you'll be glad to know, is referred to by its shorthand, OATS—can count as reconstructive surgery, and it can also be done arthroscopically. Either way, it treats cartilage injuries by taking cartilage from somewhere else in your body—somewhere that doesn't bear weight—to fill in at the injury site. Although several transplanted plugs can be used to fill up a single larger injury, this procedure works best on small injuries. A potential drawback to this type of surgery is that the harvesting leaves the places the cartilage is taken from more vulnerable to arthritis or damage.

This is a very new technique, and doctors are really just learning how to do it. As techniques get better, it will be used much more often. To date, OATS has been used primarily in patients younger than fifty (a somewhat arbitrary cut-off age established as researchers selected the patients they felt were most likely to show a benefit), though it certainly promises to be useful for patients older than that. OATS is an option for people with osteoarthritis, and surface plugs may be used after a compression fracture is repaired or a chip is removed.

Doctors are also closing in on being able to handle larger injuries this way. As it stands, patients generally make a full recovery in about six months.

ACL repair

Done as reconstructive surgery or arthroscopically, surgery on anterior cruciate ligaments (ACL) is becoming increasingly common, even while the practice of other types of surgery is decreasing. This is the injury that women and teenage girls are between two and eight times more likely to get than their male counterparts. It is especially likely to show up in athletes participating in sports that require a lot of jumping and twisting, such as basketball, skiing and soccer, and can end an athlete's season—or even career—prematurely. Surgery to repair a torn ACL, and the rehab required afterward, can cost up to thirty-five thousand dollars and take as long as six months to recover from.

For very active people, surgery may be the way to go. But if you do mostly walking, and not a lot of jumping, you may be able to live with a bad ACL, depending on the extent of the injury. Anyone who injures their ACL should wait at least a few weeks before having surgery, to let other ligaments heal and inflammation subside: You'll get better results in the end, and an easier time with rehab. Immediately following ACL injury, you'll need RICE or PRICE the first day or two, and may want to use analgesics as well. NSAIDs are controversial, as they can interfere with the immediate healing process (though they don't seem to have an impact on long-term results). Braces, too, have as many detractors as defenders because they can provide some stability, limit rotation and protect against too much strain, and can at first relieve pain and swelling; but prolonged use can stop muscles from working at their most efficient and may encourage you to be more vigorously active than you should be in the early aftermath of an injury. You do want to stay active though, at least after the first day or two, and should start working with a physical therapist to strengthen your muscles and get back your full range of motion. After all that, you may find you're doing fine, and decide to forgo surgery. There's no time limit, so you could always change your mind later if you develop problems you can't live with.

ACL surgery is not right for the youngest patients (although rates of ACL tears are increasing in school-age kids). They will be better off waiting until they have pretty much gained their full height and their skeleton has matured, so as to avoid the risk of damaging bones' growth plates.

Joint replacement

Joint replacement, in which all or part of the knee joint is replaced with an artificial one, is the last line of defense, used when damage is severe and less drastic approaches haven't provided relief. You'll be left with impressive scars from relatively large incisions, and more importantly, you'll often require an extended recovery. On top of that, the replacement may last only about fifteen years, so you may have to face the whole thing over again down the road. It is a good idea to, at the very least, put off replacement until you are at least fifty-five or sixty, to lessen the chances you'll need a second surgery when you are nearing eighty. (The idea is to die with the first replacement!) Another reason to wait is that the technology is changing so quickly that next month or next year the surgery may be easier and better.

Surgeons perform about two hundred thousand knee replacements each year in this country, and for many people it is a "miracle," even if a miracle that requires quite a bit of recovery.

This book can help you avoid being one of those statistics. But if your best efforts aren't sufficiently healing and you do decide you need a knee replacement, this program will make the process as gentle on you as possible. This is just what happened with one of my patients, Ella. She had years of relief following this program, but ultimately did need surgery. Not only did she manage to put off the surgery as long as possible without restricting her activities, but she went into the surgery strong and almost pain-free. That made the surgery as easy as possible, helped her recover speedily and well, and ensured the best possible long-term results.

Ella

Ella's knees were really ugly. Swollen. Deformed. Stiff. And very, very painful. Some days she could barely walk. Her doctor told her flat out she needed new knees. But Ella was dead set against surgery, so she started looking for a new doctor who would work with her on alternatives to going under the knife. When she finally made her way to my office, her history and physical confirmed severe osteoarthritis in the knees. The cartilage that should have been cushioning and protecting the bones that come together at the knee, keeping them moving smoothly against each other, was severely dried out and cracked. That left the bones rubbing against each other, causing irritation and inflammation—and ugly, swollen, deformed, painful and stiff knees.

Ella also had experienced changes to the bones themselves. The kind of irritation Ella had in her knees can stimulate new bone to form in abnormal shapes and in inappropriate places, causing significant irregularities in the surface of the bone, preventing the smooth glide of one part of the joint over the other, and causing increased pain and decreased mobility. Still, as long as there is some cartilage left, cartilage damage is usually reversible with nothing more complicated than excellent nutrition, reduced stress to the joint, and better knee mechanics. (These strategies might also help with the bad bony changes, but they are less effective there than in the cartilage.)

In taking her history, I also learned that Ella was a very fearful person, constantly worried by many of life's issues. The weight of her fears was literally wearing her down. I explained to Ella what foods she should eat (and not eat) to reduce inflammation—most importantly including lots of fish, nuts and berries, and eliminating sugar and simple, refined carbohydrates—and suggested some supplements, including glucosamine, chondroitin, fish oils, calcium, magnesium, and some trace minerals, as well as some anti-inflammatory herbs from both Eastern and Western traditions. I also taught her a few simple exercises to strengthen the muscles in her thighs, lower legs, pelvis and hips. Ella also learned to recognize and address her fears in more productive ways, and she learned to believe that life was good.

Ella came in for a follow-up visit two months later. Her knees were still swollen and, in fact, still ugly. But most of the pain and stiffness had stopped! Her arthritis hadn't gone away, but it no longer impinged on her life. Her knees bent easily, and she walked with no problem. In fact, she wanted to know if it was okay to start taking an exercise class, something she hadn't felt up to in years. (I gave her the green light.) She said her whole outlook had improved without the nagging pain or the nagging fear.

Four years later, Ella did have one of her knees replaced. Her pain was no longer so well controlled, and it was starting to interfere with the exercise workout she loved so much. She was concerned her pain would progress far enough to cause a limp, which could then affect the other knee. I'm happy to report that after surgery she was up and around again quickly—walking alone outdoors in about three weeks—and remains completely pain-free, which I attribute to her continuing with the steps that helped her in the years prior to surgery.

Emerging Treatments and Techniques

Most of what mainstream medicine calls upon, even its most whiz-bang technologies, is about relieving symptoms only (except, for example, surgeries that fix torn menisci or ligaments). But more and more, the talk is starting to turn to changing the disease process itself. (Of course, there's still knee pain that doesn't result from disease and the fact that prevention is the best strategy of all, but still, progress is progress!) This section looks at some of the most promising techniques on the horizon.

ALLOGRAFT MENISCAL TRANSPLANTATION

This technique trades your troubled meniscus for a healthy one from a cadaver. Besides addressing problems with the meniscus, this approach may also help with some cases of OA. It seems to stop the progression of disease, and studies show that 85 percent of patients can expect satisfactory results, although the new meniscus may tear more easily than the original. (The same procedure done with an artificial meniscus has, to date, been much less successful.)

CYCLOOXYGENASE-INHIBITING NITRIC OXIDE DONORS

These are basically the ultimate antioxidants, and currently a huge area of interest in mainstream medicine for everything from knee pain to preventing heart attacks. These anti-inflammatory agents may make even the safest NSAIDs obsolete; studies investigating their effectiveness and safety are currently underway. With any luck, they'll turn out to work best in their all-natural state—with no side effects.

PROLOTHERAPY

Prolotherapy involves injecting an irritant solution into a ligament to stimulate tissue repair and growth. While this technique has been around for at least fifty years (as a standard treatment for spider veins and hemorrhoids, where it is known as sclerotherapy), and so is actually way beyond the experimental stage, some doctors have never heard of it as a treatment for knee pain, and a limited number of them perform it. But you can read about it in the medical journals, including the most mainstream of them from time to time, and the American College of Orthopedics, the American Academy of Osteopathy and the American Osteopathic Association maintain lists of recommended prolotherapy practitioners.

The idea is that the irritant causes inflammation, and that stress on the cells makes the body release immune system proteins, spurs multiplication of repair cells in the tissue affected, and increases chemicals that encourage growth. (Sometimes, prolotherapy includes injecting those "growth factors" directly, or other chemicals that stimulate those growth factors.) Tissue built this way isn't scar tissue, which normally forms when the body is healing an injury, but normal, healthy tissue.

Prolotherapy is useful in osteoarthritis, ligament strains, loose joints, hypermobile joints, sprains and strains.

AUTOLOGOUS CHONDROCYTE IMPLANTATION (ACI)

ACI uses biotechnology to repair damaged knee cartilage. Surgeons take healthy cartilage cells (chondrocytes) from other parts of the patient's body, where healthy tissue exists, and grow them in the lab for a few weeks until they have millions of cells to work with (having started with perhaps 250,000). They then inject them right into the injured cartilage during surgery. It's a bit like repairing potholes in the road, though it is the knee joint that gets resurfaced.

The process has been proven to repair cartilage defects and, in some cases, even regenerate new tissue, and appears to be both long lasting and relatively safe. And the chance of the body rejecting the tissue is much lower than with tissue from other sources (both synthetic and from cadavers).

Wouldn't it be great to be able to simply inject something into a sore knee that would make the body produce its own cartilage—without having to cut you? This is what I believe is coming down the pike. We're already doing it, in fact, albeit in limited ways in small areas. So although I don't expect this to solve all knee problems or replace all knee surgery, this is definitely the wave of the future. I'm excited at the prospect of what is to come as this approach grows more practical, so bear with me if I dwell on it a bit longer than on some other topics.

ACI is most often done for injuries in which the cartilage inside the joint has been cracked or torn, though it can address other conditions as well, such as osteochondritis dissecans (see page 36). ACI is particularly helpful in cases in which the cartilage covering the bone has worn away; however, it is not suitable for severe OA or in cases in which there is significant bone loss because it only covers small focal areas. ACI does protect against developing arthritis in an injured joint, and the hope is that this technique will eventually be workable on old injuries—and even applied to simply stop "normal" aging of the knee. Autologous implantation can currently be done only over relatively small areas, though technology will probably improve on this point soon. For now, on larger areas, it is more common to use cadaver cartilage instead (see section on OATS, page 73).

Doctors began performing ACI more than a decade ago, and the FDA officially approved it in 1996. By 2002, it had been done 5,400 times—25 percent of them in the last year. Studies show up to 90 percent of patients improve significantly with ACI—results which have held up even in the longest lasting studies (ten years). Among the first one hundred patients to have it done in this country, 79 percent were able to go about their daily lives afterward with no pain, participating in light work and sports right up to the end of the study (five years). There's a small risk of the seal applied over the implanted cells tearing, necessitating another operation, but for the most part, ACI has proven quite successful. Larger studies are underway but not yet completed, as are studies comparing variations in technique.

ACI does require a rigorous course of physical therapy, and it'll be more than a year until you're ready to run, hit the basketball court, or do anything that will likely twist your knee. However, you will be swimming or biking much sooner than that, though not until you finish about eight weeks on crutches.

ACI avoids some of the risk of OATS (see page 73), such as increased risk of injury and of developing arthritis, because only one small (perhaps raisin-sized) sample must be extracted. ACI does have a longer recovery period than OATS, because you have to allow time to let the new cartilage cells grow. The current goal is for new, healthy cartilage to grow within a year. Experts are working on shortening both that growth period and the necessary rehab period, as well as figuring out ways to make the whole thing less invasive. For now, count on two big scars, from the initial "harvest" of cells as well as the actual surgery.

Because ACI would normally be attempted only after less drastic measures have failed, it is sometimes possible to take a sample of cells during earlier procedures and keep them in cold storage. It is probably smart to do this if you are even contemplating this procedure. If you ultimately want to grow and implant them, you'll at least avoid an additional surgery just to get the initial cells.

Tissue from cadavers can also be used in similar ways to your own cells grown in a lab, though that approach recently garnered some very bad publicity when a patient died after receiving improperly sterilized cadaver tissue that turned out to be harboring a deadly bacteria. There can also be a chance of the body rejecting the tissue.

Researchers are refining the technique, looking at using cells from outside donors, creating synthetic surfaces on which to implant cells (to improve the way they stick), and injecting cells in a fluid form that congeals inside the knee when certain wavelengths of light are applied.

It costs twelve thousand dollars just to grow the new cells. The growth factor used belongs to a particular laboratory in this country— meaning there is just one place you can have the cells grown in this country—so don't expect competition to drive the price down any time soon. The surgery itself costs just as much. And your insurance may not cover any of this. If you fight to try to get coverage, be sure to point out that this will prevent the need for a knee replacement, with all the attendant costs.

STEM CELLS

Stem cells isolated from relatively easily extracted fat tissue in the knee have been coaxed with hormones, vitamins and growth factor to grow into cartilage (or other types of cells), promising an easier way to create healthy cartilage in damaged knees. For now, this is a great concept, and much more research needs to be done.

RADIO WAVES

Radio waves have been used in arthroscopy to shrink collagen in anterior cruciate ligaments, shortening the fibers to tighten the ligaments and stabilize the joint. Early studies got the best results in only about half the patients, though when the procedure worked, it lasted as long as the study (over twenty months). This approach is currently of limited use, though more research could expand upon its promise. For now, it is most useful for acute ACL injuries.

SPACERS

Spacers implanted at the base of the thumb in arthritic patients in Swedish studies have been shown to spur growth of new healthy tissue as the device degrades over time. The Swedish biotech firm that pioneered this technique expects European Union approval to treat arthritis of the thumb this way shortly. More to the point, it already has the go-ahead in Europe to market similar biodegradable implants for the knee aimed at repairing torn ligaments, for which it will probably apply to the U.S. FDA in 2003. This is a good idea that has been around for a long time, but none of the implementations so far has borne out its promise. Perhaps this will be the material that works out, but if not, I expect research will continue in this area and will eventually turn up the right approach.

GROWTH FACTORS

Growth factors—proteins that stimulate cell growth—stimulate new growth in meniscal cells, providing an interesting possibility for future treatments in the meniscus and beyond. Imagine a few cells being prompted to grow faster and in greater numbers, healing large defects as easily as healing a cut on your finger.

GENE THERAPY

Gene therapy may also prove useful in the knee, whether through putting the genetic information you want expressed into the cells you want to affect, repairing joint damage, or replacing injured tissue. This might involve stem cells (if we can get past all the unnecessary controversy about this work), injecting DNA to stimulate new tissue growth, or some other avenue we haven't dreamed up yet. But I think what makes the most sense of all will be preventive genetics: figuring out how to stop a disease coded for in your genes from getting expressed.

SYNTHETIC LIGAMENTS

Synthetic ligaments are being investigated, though to date, the results have not kept up with similar procedures using human tissue.

Keep On Trying Till You Get It Right

If you've been to specialists and they can't find anything wrong and tell you there's nothing to be done to stop your knee pain, don't give up. *No one needs to live with knee pain.* Even if your first encounters with the medical system are unhelpful and a diagnosis can't be made, there is much to be done to relieve your pain. The program in this book shows you the options beyond the numerous standard approaches of conventional medicine. Excellent nutrition, smart exercise, postural corrections and mind-body techniques, for starters, can do wonders for your knees, and the upcoming chapters will walk you through what you need to know. A great team is half the battle, so keep trying to find medical professionals you can work with.

PREVENTION IS KEY

Your best bet is, of course, to prevent knee pain and injury in the first place. Before we get into more detail in the following chapters about what you can do to protect your knees—starting today—here's a quick overview of the roads you'll be going down:

- Maintain a healthy weight to avoid overstressing your joints. Obesity also increases the risk of degenerative conditions such as osteoarthritis. In fact, studies show that losing just ten pounds cuts your risk of osteoarthritis in half.

- Take it slowly when starting any new exercise routine, and increase intensity or duration gradually.

- Stretch before and after you exercise, especially the quadriceps muscles on the front of the thigh and the hamstrings on the back.

- Strengthen your leg muscles—all of them. The lateral and medial quads are just as important as the anterior (front) quads, which tend to get the most emphasis in most casual conditioning routines.

- Wear quality, well-fitting shoes that are in good condition and are appropriate to whatever activity you are doing, especially when exercising. This is important for maintaining proper leg alignment as well as good balance. If you have flat feet or feet that roll inward or other mechanical foot problems, look into wearing special shoe inserts (orthotics).

- Follow an anti-inflammatory and highly nutritious diet.

- Learn to productively manage your stress. If you can't decrease the input of stress, then adjust your responses, emotional or physical, to it.

- Don't ignore or try to suppress emotional upset.

- Keep your hormones in proper balance.

- Find your ideal posture—and use it.

3

Stand Up Straight: Improving Body Mechanics to Beat Knee Pain

O K, so standing up straight isn't always as easy as it sounds. But your mother was right in emphasizing the importance of good posture. The knee does not exist in its own little universe, but rather as an integral part of the anatomical, physiological, psychological and biochemical systems of your entire body. All the parts of your body are intimately connected. When your knee hurts, the problem usually isn't just in your knee.

Unfortunately, old habits—especially unconscious ones, or ones you *thought* were good—can be the source of your knee pain. Part of the problem might also be right there in your genes—how your body is put together. Fortunately, there are ways to compensate for any and all of that.

Like walking with a book on your head, it's all a matter of balance:

balanced muscle tone, balanced muscle usage, balanced nutrition, and, the focus of this chapter, balanced body mechanics—which seems just right for a joint so critical to your balance.

This is where my degree comes in handy: "D.O."—doctor of osteopathy. The emphasis of my education was on treating the whole person; I practice holistic medicine. It means that in addition to essentially the same four years of medical school that M.D.s receive, I also have additional expertise in the musculoskeletal system and the biomechanics of the body. Partly this means I sometimes do manipulations and adjustments with my patients as part of their treatment; but more important, when it comes to the knees, is having the simple awareness that how the body fits together, and how it moves, are integral to good health. Being a doctor of osteopathy means I look at the individual from a whole person perspective.

Some parts of your body get more force and more stress applied to them than others, depending on what kinds of demands are made on them. If you don't have good posture, the physical forces applied to your knees are either too harsh or in the wrong places or direction—or all of these. Something as unconscious as how you stand or walk could be part of the problem. Fixing the mechanics of the knee itself is only half the battle. You also need to fix the overall structure and mechanics of your body.

Lou

Lou runs the marathon every year. She trains carefully for months before-hand. But in the last several years, following the same old reliable training regimen, she invariably tweaks her back at about the sixteen-mile-run part of the training cycle. Then her knee starts hurting, and she becomes unable to run without pain. She self-refers to physical therapy, and her physical therapist (PT) does her best to get her through to the big run. The recent marathons have been painful, and in fact, she'd been unable to finish the last two years.

So this year, as she was gearing up to the sixteenth mile, Lou came to me with the beginning of leg and back pain. She could still run, but it was starting to hurt. A quick exam revealed that her sacrum wasn't level and that her spine had an abnormal curve to the side (scoliosis). Because she insisted on doing the marathon, we went into a crisis mode of quick-fix. So I quickly leveled her sacrum by prescribing a lift in one shoe, improving the mechanics of her entire lower body and lessening the strain on her knee and calf. I also recommended she have manipulative therapy and physical therapy.

With nothing more invasive than that, she sailed through her entire train-ing program with no injury this time around. She ran pain-free up to and through the marathon. Next year, she's aiming for a personal best. I think she can do it, too. By then she will have trained her body to stand truly up-right and the new postural habits will have become her "normal," which means not only that she will run without pain but also that the same training will produce better and better results.

Posture = Gravity vs. Structure

You have a certain structure—bones, muscles, tendons, ligaments—that holds you up, and certain forces—such as gravity—that pull you down. The sum of all those forces results in what we call posture. There are other variables, as in the depressed person who slouches, or someone who is on guard and so sits rigidly, using all his or her energy to hold the body a certain way. You can't alter gravity, so structure and those other variables are what we work on when something needs to change.

Your posture is the point of balance or equilibrium reached when you deal with the many forces acting on your body. Prime among them is gravity, which pulls down on you unrelentingly. The physical structure of your body is the resisting force holding you up. It is always a struggle, and gravity always has the upper hand. Gravity never runs out of energy or gets tired, so it is important to make the structure as strong and resilient as possible so you can offset and balance the effects of gravity.

There are many different ways a person can be out of balance. If you have one leg even just a little shorter than the other, and your body doesn't compensate in good ways, you'll list to that side as gravity pulls you down, and you will almost always develop scoliosis in the opposite direction in an attempt to balance out the forces. If your pelvis tilts backward, your head and shoulders will round forward to strike an uneasy balance. And so on. Your body does all it can to keep your eyes level with the horizon in both the side-to-side and front-to-back planes (which is crucial for the way in which our various senses are able to work together, e.g., your ears and eyes have the same horizon so you don't get vertigo). To that end, we compensate for the downward pull of gravity in a variety of ways. Your center of gravity—the weight-bearing line that results from the balancing of all these forces—when properly balanced, spreads stresses around so all your joints can share in absorbing the force applied, so that no one joint (for instance, the knee) becomes overstressed. But when the structure is off, the center of gravity is off and we may develop problems. An example of this is the Leaning Tower of Pisa; as the foundation sinks more on one side than the other, the whole tower bends more and various floors bend more than other floors, depending upon their individual strengths.

Good body mechanics manifests in good posture, and vice versa. To visualize what normal posture would be, imagine a weighted string hung from your ear. To someone looking at you from the side, it should look like the string passes through the center of your ear, your shoulder, the curve of your lower back (actually, the center of the third lumbar vertebrae), the front third of the top of your sacrum, your hip, the outside of your knee, and the center of the outside ankle bone. With all of these landmarks lined up, the body is best able to support and distribute the weight from front to back.

Check yourself out from the front as well. Your feet should be square on the ground, your knees pointing straight ahead, your pelvis and shoulders level, and your head rising straight above your shoulders (not tilted to one side or the other). Your legs should look the same length and symmetrically muscular, and your knees should be the same height off the ground. All this balances your weight from side to side. If you draw a line on the ground and stand toe-to-toe to it, your knees,

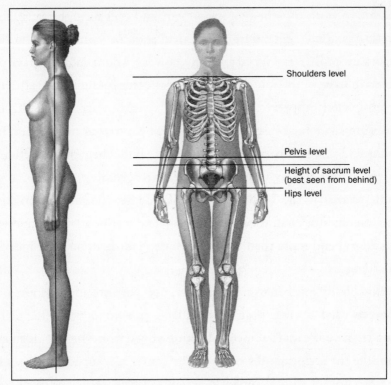

Shoulders level

Pelvis level

Height of sacrum level
(best seen from behind)

Hips level

hip and shoulders should also be square to that line: That balances you in the rotational plane.

Your sacrum (the base of your spine and part of the pelvis bones) is your body's weight-bearing center, and your alignment will fall into place around it, ideally, in the straight line we're talking about. But if one landmark is out of line, it will most probably pull out others in a kind of compensation (known as the compensatory mechanism). If your shoulders are rounded, for instance, you will probably see that your upper body is leaning backward a bit, putting your shoulders behind your sacrum. You will also probably notice that your head will be bent forward in front of your shoulders. You do this compensation in order to equalize the weight in front of and behind the weight-bearing lines we described earlier. While you are balancing your weight, with a part of you in front of the midline and a part of you behind the midline, this is still undesirable because it creates a very inefficient mechanical structure that stresses each of the joints, resulting in damage. This awkward balance redistributes weight to your knees and feet, and not for the better.

If it doesn't come naturally, you should practice getting yourself into alignment. Yes, just stand there. (Or sit there, in which case your weight should be even on both ischial ["sit"] bones, and your shoulders should be square, with your head directly above them, smack in the middle both from side to side and from front to back.) You might want to get someone to take your picture, with as few clothes on as you can manage, so you can study your posture yourself. Be sure to get views from the front, back and side.

If finding good posture doesn't happen with ease, it can almost always be made to happen with a proper training program. I find the best results come from combining osteopathic manipulative therapy with appropriate physical therapy. At home you can improve your balance with large exercise balls such as those sold under the brand name Physioball (and a book or tape to suggest exercises) and work on your alignment, balance and strength through books or videos of Pilates, qi gong, tai chi or yoga workouts.

Of course you need good posture when you are in motion as well as when you are stationary, and the best alignment at any given moment depends on what you are doing. Think of the way expert tennis players, golfers, baseball players and many other athletes stand when they are ready for action: legs shoulder-width apart, knees slightly bent, weight centered over the balls of their feet. They are in balance, and are ready to move quickly and to absorb impact. That's why it looks so effortless when the pros do what they do. They need a minimum of effort because balance allows for efficiency, and vice versa; it doesn't hurt that their muscles are also strong. (It is worth noting that pro athletes these days have individualized training programs that often as not include nutrition, supplements and sport psychologists right along with gym work and practice.)

No matter what activity you are engaged in, as long as you are standing, your knees should be relaxed and slightly bent. Don't stand or walk with locked knees. You need that slight bend to keep springiness in your knees, to allow them to adapt to changing terrain. Imagine walking up stairs with your knees locked. Besides being difficult, think of what abnormal motions you would create for your feet, ankles, hips, spine, shoulders and neck. That would create wear and tear in abnormal directions, resulting in damage to the soft tissues (ligaments, tendons and cartilage) and, in the long run, the bones—OA.

If you are not convinced that your posture is perfect in all planes, you might want to get a professional evaluation from an osteopathic physician or other experienced health-care provider. It is true that sore knees may affect the way you move—but it is equally true that the way you move can set you up for sore knees. An expert opinion can help you sort out the chicken/egg aspects of your situation. An osteopathic physician, for example, would be checking your alignment as well as your gait and stride, the way your feet and ankles move, how well your body bears weight, your strength, the sequence of muscle firing, the length of your legs and your pelvic tilt, among other things. A yoga instructor or other bodywork expert may also be able to help. But just having a friend or partner stand at your side, facing you, and drawing this imaginary line can let you know if you are carrying your head too far forward, rounding your shoulders, rocking back on your feet, or whatever. You'll soon understand that "standing up straight" isn't always the right image: It can lead to throwing your shoulders back, hyperextending your back or otherwise getting out of alignment.

Problematic Posture

Abnormal or troublesome posture can be the result of birth defects, developmental problems, malnutrition (like a condition such as rickets), trauma (small or large, physical or emotional), a poorly balanced exercise regimen, and even psychological upset. You may also carry yourself in a way that is actually causing pain thanks to habits you aren't even conscious of.

Part of the problem is simply the way the human body is put together. The knees really took a beating when humans began walking upright—no more four sets of knuckles on the ground to equally carry the weight! Perhaps as we continue to evolve over millions more years, we'll move beyond this beta version and perfect the design. (Not that that does us any good right now.) Who knows?—while we wait for Mother Nature to solve the issue, maybe we'll get comfortable, smart shoes designed in some way to help us out.

It may be that your anatomy is such that the angles your bones meet at, the orientation of your kneecap, or the "looseness" or "tightness" of your ligaments or tendons are causing your knee pain. But studies show that not all people with any given anatomical pattern usually associated with knee pain experience any knee pain. On the other hand, many, many people *without* anatomical "abnormalities" do experience knee pain. Something more is going on than simply bad design.

More important than how your body is actually put together is how you use it. This determines how much stress (or "mechanical load") is put on your anatomy, whatever it looks like. Whether the stress is short and high-impact, as when jumping off stairs, or low-key but cumulative, as when walking on cement floors all day, mechanical load can cause structural and cartilage damage, such as wearing away of the cartilage, straining the ligaments and/or tendons, and exaggerating scoliosis, among other things. Imagine what would happen if you tried to carry a one-hundred-pound box on one shoulder. Your body would respond by going into crisis mode—your head would list one way, as would your shoulders, hips, knees and ankles. Further imagine if you had structural problems, and various compensations for them, to begin with. And imagine the long-term effects of these chronic strains if you were to do this every day. And think of your poor, poor knees. Minimizing and controlling mechanical load—often through postural or musculoskeletal adjustments, or just training your muscles to optimally deal with the variances of your body's structure—is key to treating knee pain.

Unconscious musculoskeletal patterns in your body often play a role in knee pain. Skeletal asymmetry is a common culprit. If your pelvis isn't level, for example, it puts uneven loads on the two sides of your body, especially at the low back, hip, knee, foot and ankle—any or all of which can cause knee pain. If your feet roll inward ("pronation") or your knees tend to bow outward, you're likely to feel that in your knees as well. And those are just the most popular entries on the list of specific postures that cause trouble.

Fortunately, they can be corrected relatively simply—once they are properly diagnosed—with strengthening exercises (see Chapter Ten), postural training such as that mentioned above, proprioceptive training, and neuromuscular reeducation, which we'll cover in Chapters Six and Ten. Proprioceptive training such as balance and coordination exercises teaches the body to know where all its parts are in relation to each other at any given moment. An example of a situation in which proprioceptive training is important would be when I see patients who are standing crooked. When I ask them to stand straight, they inevitably say that they are. Their normal is "crooked," and this is what they learn to work around.

This abnormal postural compensation must be addressed before you begin to strengthen your muscles, or you will just encourage the muscles to keep making the same errors—only more so. You must learn a new "better" normal before you begin to strengthen muscles. Strengthening in abnormal posture only reinforces the abnormal patterns.

Neuromuscular reeducation is teaching the muscles to work correctly by normalizing patterns of brain to muscle communication, involving things like sequence of muscle firing and a balanced strength program. It's like learning to use your hand or leg again after a stroke has disrupted communication between the brain and the muscles, except that you are breaking old habits before you learn new strength techniques.

After all that, if you still need it, you can get custom-designed lifts in your shoes (orthotics) to help push you in the correct direction.

COMMON STRUCTURAL PROBLEMS

Women have a good number of unique structural issues that impact the knees: Women's wider hips cause their thigh bones to angle in, which in turn causes their knees to angle out; the shape of women's kneecaps are different from men's; women's kneecaps track differently than do men's; women stand more erect than men; women generally have stronger quads than hamstrings. All of these variables alter the mechanical forces in play, and contribute to understanding why women are more prone to so many knee problems.

Of course there are a range of other structural issues, some of them anatomical, some more habitual—and some a combination of both. Here we will look at the most common.

There are good ways to compensate for all of them, though the first step is always the same: Figure out where your body is out of good alignment, and why. The ideal is to get as close to perfect posture, in as close to perfect balance, as possible, whatever you have to do to get there.

Exaggerated Q angle

The way the bones of the upper and lower leg angle in to each other at the knee, known as the Q angle, is distinctly different in women when compared to men.

If you drew a line from the outside front of the pelvis down to the kneecap, and another line from the middle of the ankle, in the front, up to and over the kneecap, the angle at which they intersect is known as the Q angle (see illustration on page 99). Because they tend to have wider pelvises and their knees angle inward, women tend to have more

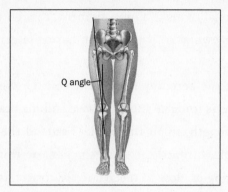

dramatic Q angles than men. That in and of itself isn't a problem, but if the Q angle is too exaggerated on anyone it can interfere with the smooth tracking of the kneecap as it moves over the leg bones, causing chondromalacia patella, patellofemoral syndrome, or ligament strain—in any event, knee pain!

An exaggerated Q angle is always a problem if there is asymmetrical strength in the thigh muscles, which is quite common. The kneecap is drawn up by all four of the quadriceps muscles. If there is an imbalance in the four muscles, the kneecap will be pulled more to the left or the right (away from the weaker muscle), which will also cause pain. A larger than average Q angle puts you at higher risk of patellofemoral syndrome.

"Normal" Q angle should be fifteen to twenty degrees or less (ten to eighteen degrees or less in men). However, whatever your Q angle, treatment is going to address the problems it causes—it's not going to change the Q angle. So if you have a higher Q angle, that may explain the problem, but treatment means learning to compensate better.

An accurate measurement of your Q angle is probably in order—ask a physical therapist, orthopedist, osteopath or other knowledgeable medical professional to make a measurement, though you can make an estimate on your own as to whether you have a larger than normal Q angle.

In any event, the best way to prevent your Q angle from causing you any problems is to make sure you have and maintain correctly balanced muscle strength, in all the muscles around the knee joint, and correct foot, ankle, hip and sacral mechanics. By this I mean having every joint working as close to mechanically correct as is possible. Remember that any one joint moving incorrectly can—and most likely will—cause the other joints to be stressed and possibly even damaged. You should consider getting a professional to help you evaluate and correct these problems.

Unequal leg lengths

Almost a quarter of all Americans actually have a difference of one centimeter or more in the length of their legs; about one in one thousand have enough of a difference to require a corrective device, such as a lift or orthotic. (Still, those devices are too often diagnosed when the real problem is a sacrum that isn't level; see page 102.) In the rare event that the difference in length is drastic enough, surgery to lengthen or shorten one leg or the other may be required.

A healed hip or leg fracture from a childhood injury can result in different leg lengths. In fact, any old injury that occurred during bone-growing years (up through sixteen to eighteen in women) could interrupt or slow bone growth and cause some asymmetry. Hip dysplasias (a dislocation of the hip seen in babies and children), congenital malformation, and developmental or nutritional problems can also cause legs of different lengths.

Assessing your leg length starts with a simple examination, although your doctor may order a standing-up X ray (officially, "erect lumbosacral postural studies") or other diagnostic test if he or she suspects a significant discrepancy. The classic clinical assessment, however, involves having you stand on various sized blocks until your *sacrum* is level. The doctor can then prescribe a lift of the same height as the block that straightens you out when you stand on it.

There's a number of problems with that approach, however. First, even when physicians measure carefully with their hands, they are wrong more than half the time. So wrong, in fact, that sometimes it is really the *other* leg that's actually shorter. Second, except in acute cases (after surgery or a fracture), what should be corrected is not the length of the legs but the sacrum's inability to compensate for the leg-length discrepancy. Nobody is perfectly symmetrical, but the sacrum is supposed to be able to make amends.

The only absolutely reliable way to get an accurate measurement is with an X ray done standing up, using a very specific protocol. The only way to have accurate X ray film is to be sure the floor is level and the films are exactly parallel and perpendicular to the floor, so you need to go to a practice set up to do this sort of thing. You should stand with your feet shoulder-width apart, with your arms at your sides and your knees straight, in your normal posture.

If you do fracture a leg or hip bone, or have a surgery that results in one leg being shorter than the other, this should immediately be addressed by whatever means (i.e., a lift) to correct it so that you don't develop compensatory problems such as scoliosis.

In any event, if you do need a lift, it should be tailored to you. Don't be tempted to buy a ready-made one over the counter in the drugstore. A generic lift like that may bring you some relief quite quickly, but may well start or encourage other bad compensatory habits and create new pains.

If you have one of those acute conditions resulting from surgery or a bone break, you will get a lift to fix it all at once. But if length discrepancy originates from something else and is a more chronic problem, you have to correct it gradually. For example, you might start out with a three millimeter lift, and increase it two millimeters every month until reaching the desired height. Differences of more than twelve millimeters get more complicated, and are likely to involve adjusting the height of the opposite sole. In any event, your doctor will use a formula integrating many variables (including your age, how long you've had the problem, and more) to determine how quickly to correct sacral height differences. In my practice, I see a patient every two weeks after a new lift to do manipulations, and I adjust the lift if necessary every four weeks, until all measurements are correct. I usually find that by doing manipulations and physical therapy, the patient winds up with a lift about one half the height of the uneven sacral difference.

Uneven sacrum

As we discussed, many of us have uneven legs, and a normally functioning sacrum can compensate for about a one-quarter to one-half inch difference. A shorter leg is only a problem when the sacrum can't compensate for it, because of anatomical variances in shape, mechanical failures (i.e., loose ligaments), postural problems or nutritional lack. To fix the problem, we must correct the sacrum's inability to compensate.

A nonlevel sacrum results in abnormal forces on knees, ankles and hips. Among other things, if your sacrum is canted, there's increased stress on your knee, especially when you walk or run. This results in pain due to mechanical stress. An uneven sacrum is one of the underlying causes of iliotibial band friction syndrome. This is a frequent cause of knee pain in runners and other athletes who run or jump a lot (as described in Chapter One). With the pelvis lower on one side than the other resulting in uneven hips, the awkward displacement of stress on the knee can result in inflammation and pain. This is also among the most frequent causes of scoliosis, which puts strain and stress on your knees too.

Bowleggedness

About half of all people with osteoarthritis are at least a little bow-legged (though they can also be knock-kneed; see below). The bow-leggedness means the knee wears down asymmetrically, with more strain on the inside of the knee than the outside, meaning uneven wear and tear on cartilage and ligaments and menisci. Proprioception training and neuromuscular reeducation can help a great deal, as can lifts and orthotics.

Knock-kneed/pigeon-toed

This condition is also common in people with osteoarthritis. With the knees tilting inward toward each other and the feet pointing toward each other, one side of the knee gets much more strain, and wear and tear, than the other side; when your joint loses its ability to compensate for this, you begin to get pain and damage. The poor mechanics result in wear and tear on the joint, increasing the risk of developing osteoarthritis.

Here again, proprioception training and neuromuscular reeducation can help a great deal, and the younger you are when you start, the better. Physical therapy, braces and sometimes even surgery can be used to change the angle of the knee and the way force is directed on the joint.

Foot pronation

If your ankles roll inward, your knee is forced to bow out a bit, ligaments get thrown off of level, and the pelvis tilts as well, resulting once again in poor weight distribution over the joints and too much force applied unevenly to the knee. Pronation predisposes you to patellofemoral syndrome. Professional orthotics or lifts can help your foot stay properly placed.

High heels

As you might imagine, walking around on the balls of your feet all day—like any abnormal stance—is tough on your knees. Any time you step out in heels over two inches high, you place seven times your weight onto the ball of the foot, once again concentrating a lot of force on one point rather than sharing the wealth—a classic set up for knee pain. You also create a situation in which you don't straighten your knee when you walk—your weight-balancing mechanism is thrown off because you always keep your knee bent to be able to walk through your next step. You also affect muscle length, shortening the gastrics and lengthening the quads. To balance your weight now, your body has to make adjustments all the way up your leg, thigh and hip, and this results in the pelvis and sacrum having to adjust to these new forces so that your upper and lower body can maintain a functional center of gravity.

Here the solution is very simple: Lose the heels. Well, lower them, anyway. I recommend a low heel—whatever height helps you get that imaginary plumb line straight. Some people can't wear flats, some can only wear flats. Nobody can wear three- or four-inch heels everyday! Keep it to two inches or less, in well-fitting shoes with good support. And if you occasionally want to slip into a pair of high heels? Well, the better shape you are in, the less strain you will experience from each exposure; the more fragile your state, the more vulnerable you are to having a problem.

Scoliosis

There are too many causes of curvature of the spine to discuss them all here. In any case, the resulting uneven weight distribution will create structural failures in you not unlike what happened to the Leaning Tower of Pisa!

Flat feet, splayed feet and high arches

Because the foot must adjust to the center of gravity of the body above it, there is a great deal of mechanical force distributed throughout. The tiny bones and muscles of the foot take all your body weight and all of your body's force and distribute it over the length and width of your foot. This is a great deal of force and requires all the bones and muscles to work together to distribute the force in a functionally sound manner. If there are mechanical problems in the foot (when standing and, more importantly, when moving), stress and strain result. This must be evaluated by a professional who can address the foot mechanics but who will also see the foot in relationship to the knee, hip, sacrum and pelvis.

Sonya

Sonya's knee was clearly a mess. She had torn cartilage, strained and torn ligaments, and arthritis to boot. Her orthopedist said she didn't need a knee replacement, and short of that offered only a lifelong course of anti-inflammatory drugs and pain medicine. Sonya had managed to get a referral for physical therapy, but didn't think that it was really helping. She felt she got some pain relief from acupuncture.

When Sonya came to see me, we determined that her knees angled in toward each other—she was "knock-kneed"—which puts a great deal of strain on the knees. On visual examination, I discovered that her sacrum, the bone in her pelvis, was higher on one side than the other—making one leg effectively shorter than the other. Fortunately, that wasn't hard to adjust with osteopathic manipulation, and I leveled the sacrum so that with each step the same amount of force fell on the foot, knee and hip of each leg. The force was redistributed so that it wasn't all on one side, and one knee. The manipulation sessions took twenty to thirty minutes, and continued weekly over several months—a fairly typical course for a chronic problem (though simple adjustments can be done in as little as one session). I used a combination of many techniques, each designed to effect a specific correction. These, when done in the proper sequence and when supported by a coordinated and proper exercise regimen, created the desired results. Neither osteopathic manipulation nor physical therapy alone would work. Osteopathy made her straight but couldn't keep her there. PT didn't make her straight; it only strengthened her improper positions. But together they were healing.

I also recommended several supplements to Sonya, including glucosamine, collagen and collagen-forming nutrients such as amino acids, mucopolysaccharides, silica, copper, zinc, B vitamins, and omega-3 and omega-6 oils, which are anti-inflammatory. (See Chapter Nine for more information on using supplements to fight knee pain.)

"Within two months, I couldn't believe how great I felt," she says. "My knee pain—which other doctors had told me I should learn to live with—just went away. What surprised me most was that the work I needed wasn't on my knee at all."

Getting rid of—or better still, preventing—knee pain will involve an analysis of all these factors and more, to see which applies in your case. It may well require professional help to find and maintain the perfect balance for your body. It will be worth it for posture that makes you look and feel great, and protects your knees in the bargain. Plus, it will make your mother proud.

4

Hormones and Your Knees

When you have cramps or hot flashes, or are retaining water, I bet you've been heard cursing your hormones. But I bet you never considered laying your knee pain on their doorsteps. I'm here to tell you that they may well be at the root of your problem, and that getting your hormones functioning smoothly may end up healing your knees as well as any more obvious symptoms you may have.

It isn't really the hormones themselves that cause you any problems. Though you may be prone to griping about them, hormones are in fact your friends. They are critical to just about every system in your body—you wouldn't be alive without them—and necessary for vibrant good health. The trouble starts, rather, when hormones that need to work in intricate relationships with one another fall out of sync and become imbalanced.

Be warned: Hormonal imbalances or shifts take their toll on your joints as well as the rest of you. Problematic changes in hormone levels can come from many causes, including menstrual cycle, menopause, pre- or perimenopause, stress, and environmental exposure to foreign hormones (not structured like those that our bodies make) found in our food chain and pollutants, hormone replacement therapy, and some forms of birth control. Just about everything you do in your life will affect when and how your hormones fluctuate, and when they do, even small changes in the optimal orchestration of your hormones can wreak havoc on your body. One of the common results is aches and pains, including (but certainly not limited to) knee pain.

If you are low in testosterone, for example (which women do need, though in smaller amounts than men), or in cortisol (one of the hormones that helps you handle stress), you may experience muscle loss, weakness and joint pain. Problems with thyroid hormone levels, too, can cause problems in your knees, as we'll see later in this chapter. For women, however, the most common hormone linked to knee problems is estrogen, and more specifically the ratio of estrogen to progesterone, which we will discuss further later in this chapter.

You can't just keep tabs on one hormone or another to avoid or fix your knee pain (or any other problem you think is hormonally related). Hormones work in complex relationships with each other. One triggers the production, release, uptake, inhibition or destruction of another. Various hormones can be converted by the body one into the other. Keeping hormone levels in balance is crucial for good health—and avoiding knee pain—but that balance is a delicate one. In medical school, doctors are taught the primacy of the "HPA axis"—the hypothalamus, pituitary and adrenal glands—which sends signals back and forth to stimulate or reduce various hormones. In truth, there are even more glands critical to the normal ebb and flow of hormones in the body, not least of which are the thyroid and ovaries. All are strongly connected to the brain, intertwined with the neurological system as well as immunological function. No one gland can work in isolation. I think the endocrine system is the most complicated in the entire body. Even the endocrinologists I know think it is very complicated!

Consider, for example, the group known as steroid hormones (estrogen, progesterone, testosterone, cortisol and others). All of these are made from cholesterol (not the food, but the hormone you produce), and the basic chemical structure of each of them is very similar to this precursor—and so very similar to that of the others. But obviously they have very different effects on the body: I'm sure you wouldn't willingly trade your levels of estrogen and testosterone! Well, the two are chemically identical except for one hydrogen atom and one chemical bond. That's it, right there, one major difference between a man and a woman (or so one could argue). Beyond the fact that they are derived from the same source, these hormones are also made from each other. Imagine a river flowing from a spot upstream known as cholesterol to a variety of downstream ports: progesterone, DHEA, testosterone, estrogen, etc. At any port the quality or quantity of material sent to the next port can change. And when it does, ripples are felt all up and down the river; the balance between and among all the hormones shifts as well. If estrogen levels fall, progesterone may cause unpleasant symptoms. If DHEA falls, testosterone will fall and cause a low testosterone problem.

One could devote an entire book to the subject of hormone balance and how each individual can detect, achieve and/or monitor it. We've got other things to do in the rest of this book, so in this chapter I just want to give you an overview of how hormones affect women's knees, and point you on your way to learning how to rebalance your hormones with diet and supplements and, if strictly necessary, supplemental natural hormones, all in the interest of relieving knee pain (among other symptoms). Each person is different, so there's no one-size-fits-all prescription I can offer here for perfect hormone balance. But if you learn to listen to what your body is telling you, as outlined in this chapter, you'll be able to ferret out the areas you need to be concerned about, and know what avenues to pursue with your doctor.

Estrogen

Estrogen, like all steroid hormones, has anti-inflammatory effects. When estrogen is out of balance with and/or overwhelmed by other hormones, inflammation and other problems result. PMS, uncomfortable symptoms of menopause, and many other symptoms are caused by similar hormonal imbalances. It's no coincidence that knee problems flare up for so many women right around menopause—and that in younger women some studies show that knee injuries spike at certain times of the menstrual cycle when estrogen levels drop. Many experts count a low estrogen level as a risk for osteoarthritis, though that's controversial. By the same token, hormone replacement therapy has been shown to protect against developing osteoarthritis and to slow its progression.

A competing theory holds that since estrogen relaxes soft tissue and slows collagen synthesis, it can "loosen" ligaments, making joints more vulnerable to poor alignment, instability and, ultimately, injury when estrogen levels are high, as levels fluctuate during the menstrual cycle, or at menopause—or certainly, in comparison to men. Rates of knee pain and injury clearly increase after menopause. And studies done at the University of Michigan and Cincinnati Sports Medicine Clinic show that female athletes are more likely to have a knee injury while they are ovulating—that is, when their estrogen levels are at their peak.

It may be that both the anti-inflammatory and the loose ligament scenarios are true, depending on how a specific woman's body reacts to estrogen and hormone imbalance, and on the other factors contributing to knee pain for any given woman.

Just when in the menstrual cycle the danger zone for women falls, however, has yet to be firmly established. Estrogen drops dramatically premenstrually—and some studies show injuries occur disproportionately more during that same time frame. Other studies, however, associate increases in injuries with the follicular phase (during a period and the first few days after, as estrogen starts to rise), and still others with the mid-cycle ovulatory phase, when estrogen has risen and begins to fall again. To cloud matters further, women who take birth control pills (and so have more constant estrogen levels throughout their cycles) still injure their ACLs at a comparable rate to women not on the Pill.

More studies might be useful in pinning down the cyclical nature of women's vulnerability to knee injury. More to the point, however, would be to note the difficulty of tying any one effect to any one hormone. This is because the interplay of various hormones in the body is so intricate, and what's most important is not any one level but the balance between and among estrogen, progesterone, testosterone, cortisol and others.

To add to the mix, estrogen helps control sensitivity to pain, and when estrogen levels drop, perception of pain increases. This is why, for example, women react to pain differently depending on where they are in their cycle. (Progesterone and testosterone fluctuations no doubt contribute as well.) Some experts find women to be less sensitive to pain than men—except in women with low estrogen levels, whose perception of pain is generally on par with men's. Restoring estrogen levels into balance with other hormones can once again limit sensitivity to pain.

The brain produces chemicals called endorphins that mediate pain. Estrogen increases the number of sites in the brain available for the endorphins to attach to do their work. When estrogen levels are high, pain-killing endorphins are effectively more powerful. The brain can better control the response to pain—i.e., you feel less pain. (This comes in very handy in keeping the birth rate up: A woman's estrogen spikes just before delivery.)

A recent study demonstrated quite clearly how estrogen helps reduce the perception of pain by making images of chemical changes in the brain as volunteers were subjected to a painful muscle spasm when they had higher and lower levels of estrogen (at a certain point in the menstrual cycle, and using an estrogen patch). With more estrogen, the brain scans showed more endorphin activity, and volunteers reported less pain. There's every reason to believe this would work the same way where knee pain is the issue.

Low estrogen is associated with the production of inflammatory substances called cytokines, which aid and abet pain from strains, sprains, OA and other things, and interfere with muscle metabolism and function. (These inflammatory changes are always made worse when there are any other inflammatory triggers, such as allergies, toxic exposure or increased stress.)

The estrogen–knee-pain link has become more and more pronounced in recent years. Our society and culture exposes women to hugely increased levels of estrogen from sources outside their own bodies, mainly from pollutants and foods. Hormones in food given to cattle, chickens and some farm-bred fish to make them grow faster are structurally similar to estrogen, and the meat (especially organ meat), milk, cheese and eggs from the animals fed these chemicals have all kinds of excess estrogens (the absence of which is another of the benefits of organic, free-range foods). Plastics, even plastic wrap, can contaminate us with estrogen-like substances as well, as can other pollutants.

With so much excess estrogen influencing them, progesterone levels in our bodies are generally decreased relative to estrogen (and in some cases absolutely decreased), and so many women are in "estrogen dominance"—a combination of excess estrogen and deficient progesterone—an imbalance that can create all kinds of symptoms, not least of which is knee pain.

Rates of knee pain in women escalate dramatically right around menopause—which is, of course, a major shift in the way hormones are balanced in the body. Perimenopause, the phase just before menopause, actually features even more hormone hijinks and for many women brings, among other fun and enjoyable symptoms, the start of knee pain.

Other than pregnancy, perimenopause is the time of life when a woman's estrogen levels reach their highest (and sometimes their lowest) point. Perimenopause is a time of great change in hormone levels.

At perimenopause, estrogen levels are often actually *higher* than they were before perimenopause, but fluctuate much more. The symptoms of perimenopause, including night sweats, poor sleep, hot flashes, memory problems, depression and more, are not always due to low estrogen, as is commonly thought, but to the rapid change from higher to lower estrogen experienced during these fluctuations. "Lower" does not have to mean lower than normal to cause symptoms—just lower than it was before. The change in levels alone can cause problems. Furthermore, the hormonal shift brings about an imbalance between estrogen and progesterone, as well as between estrogen and the substances that result from the breakdown of estrogen and progesterone. It is these imbalances that stimulate the release of neurotransmitters and hormones that produce the all too familiar vasomotor symptoms of perimenopause and menopause, such as hot flashes, sweaty palms, tight muscles, nervousness, shakiness, agitation and migraine headaches.

Bringing all this back to joint pain, and knee pain specifically: Increased estrogen, and then the rapid change to lower levels, stimulates or enhances the activity of a certain type of white blood cell called, if you must know, polymorphonuclear leukocytes—or PNL, for those of us who like less of a mouthful. This increased PNL activity results in an increase in the release of inflammatory substances called cytokines. And the increase in these inflammation-causing cytokines can result in joint pain.

Those same cytokines, the production of which is ultimately spurred by changes in estrogen levels, can also cause many fibromyalgia-like symptoms, including fatigue, muscle aches and weakness, joint stiffness and multiple trigger points (some of which are located around the knee). Without enough energy to properly run the body, and with a decrease in proper muscle function, joints—especially the knee—will suffer.

Any foreign substances in the body, including excess hormones or hormones foreign to your body (such as estrogens from the environment that are similar but not identical to the ones your body makes), are "antigens," and the body must produce antibodies to battle them. The resulting immune complex (antibodies attached to antigens) is absorbed by the body and can cause, if not disease, then certainly symptoms—and can interfere with hormone levels. For instance, the most commonly prescribed estrogen (for hormone replacement therapy) is made from horse's urine—foreign to the human body—and is also about fifty times stronger than our own strongest estrogen; faced with this, it is very hard for the body to maintain a balance between it and all the other hormones estrogen affects.

Cartilage is most commonly affected, because the antigen proteins are very similar to the protein in cartilage. There is, after all, more protein in collagen (found in cartilage and connective tissue) than anywhere else in the body; when the body sees foreign proteins, they can look like cartilage, and when the body starts to attack the invaders, it gets its own cartilage too. (This is why rheumatoid arthritis affects the joints.) The bottom line is, having your own estrogen remain normal in both its level and its relationship to your other hormones will go a long way toward helping your knees.

Thyroid Hormones

The other common hormone link to knee pain involves thyroid hormones. Joint pain is one of the typical symptoms of low thyroid hormone levels (along with others listed in the box at the end of this chapter). Low thyroid levels can also weaken muscles and even make you lose muscle mass. The body uses the thyroid hormone T3 to control calcium movement across neuromuscular barriers, and without sufficient supplies, the muscles can't work right. Weak leg muscles, or uneven strength in your legs, is a set up for knee pain.

In addition, thyroid problems are associated with an increase in the incidence of chronic illness, including arthritis and other joint pain that may well settle in your knees. Recently published studies of older people showed that patients with the most chronic illnesses (such as high blood pressure, heart disease and arthritis) had the highest levels of thyroid antibodies and those who were the healthiest had low or no thyroid antibodies. The presence of those thyroid antibodies means the immune system perceives the thyroid gland as a foreign substance and is fighting it off. That can be associated with either high or low levels of thyroid hormone, or you could have high thyroid antibodies but normal levels of thyroid hormone. But the most important thing to know is that if you don't address the cause of those high antibody levels, eventually your hormone levels will be off; most commonly you'll become hypothyroid. Because high levels of thyroid antibodies are a sign of an autoimmune reaction, it doesn't surprise me that they often show up alongside other conditions, especially those that may also be from an autoimmune reaction.

About 85 percent of women with low thyroid levels are in that situation as a result of an autoimmune reaction. The name given to low thyroid function resulting from an autoimmune condition is Hashimoto's disease. (The other 15 percent with low thyroid levels but not Hashimoto's probably lack the nutrients to make thyroid hormone, have thyroid damage from radiation or from iodine deficiency, or have adrenal gland problems that prevent thyroid hormone from getting into the cells. The autoimmune reaction means that the body is responding to a perceived or real threat from outside. It does this by producing antibodies against the foreign invader (antigen). When the body misinterprets a cold virus antigen, for example, as thyroid or cartilage, then we produce antibodies to battle those tissues. The result is an autoimmune illness: The body is fighting off some of its own cells as if they were dangerous foreign invaders. When the antibodies the body forms to protect itself attach to the antigens, the result is what is called an immune complex. That immune complex can go from the source of the battle into the bloodstream and from there to anywhere in the body—and it has a strong affinity for cartilage in the joints, attacking it as another invader, damaging the cartilage in the course of the battle. Anytime the immune system is working overtime, as it so often is with hypothyroidism, joint pain—knee pain—is a not uncommon result.

The symptoms of Hashimoto's are the same as anyone's with low thyroid levels (see the box at the end of this chapter), with the addition of the fact that the immune complexes formed as a result of the body attacking the thyroid hormone it perceives as an unwanted invader can also affect other organs and create other diseases. Autoimmune disorders such as Hashimoto's disease *also* cause hormonal imbalance, which, as we've seen, leads to knee pain.

Alternatively, you might have all the symptoms of low thyroid, but your thyroid gland appears healthy and is producing normal levels of the hormones. That indicates that your adrenal gland is not working properly, with the result that your body can't properly absorb and use the thyroid hormone available to it. The adrenal gland plays a large part in how you handle stress, whether physical or emotional, mainly by its production of cortisone, which also decreases inflammation (just as cortisone, DHEA and adrenaline are prescribed to do).

An adrenal gland not working well (because of increased demand from chronic stress, lack of nutrients, or tumors, among other causes) has a hard time controlling inflammation, which often means knee pain. The appropriate treatment is of the adrenal gland, not the thyroid, and should relieve joint pain along with the more typical thyroid-related symptoms. The exact treatment depends on the ultimate cause of the adrenal problems, but a typical course would include stress-reduction techniques, herbs and nutrients to feed the adrenal gland, and eating along the lines suggested in this book, to decrease inflammation.

It may simply be that an autoimmune reaction that is causing you thyroid problems also causes joint pain. Or you could have a genetic predisposition toward specific autoimmune reactions, whether thyroid problems, arthritis, or anything else. It is—for various reasons—common for the body to produce an antibody against cartilage—essentially attacking the cartilage as an invader. Weakened cartilage, of course, results in knee pain.

Why cartilage is so often affected is unclear. Probably it is because there is more protein in cartilage than anywhere else in the body, and reactions to foreign proteins drive our immune response. The link is seen in many autoimmune disorders; lupus, psoriasis and rheumatoid arthritis (as distinct from the osteoarthritis we've focused on in this book) are the classic examples.

Up to 80 percent of hypothyroid patients can wind up not needing supplemental prescription thyroid hormones over the long haul, assuming we catch it early. (People with long-standing thyroid issues, or who have taken hormones for a long while, are another story.) Once we find and address the underlying cause of their immune system upset, be it parasites or a chronic bacterial or viral infection, heavy metal toxicity, or food sensitivities, their antibodies go away, and their bodies make and use sufficient thyroid hormones again. Those who do start on thyroid medicine in order to more rapidly control their symptoms are still usually able to stop or reduce their doses once the underlying problems are brought under control.

Getting the right nutrients—vitamins, minerals, herbs, EFAs, and more—can help your thyroid produce the hormones you need, when and how you need them. They can stimulate the thyroid, increasing thyroid hormones and increasing the cells' ability to use thyroid hormones as well as your body's sensitivity to them. The thyroid gland produces the thyroid hormone T4, which the body converts, outside the thyroid, into T3, which body cells respond to more than to T4. Your body needs good nutrition to help it increase T3, change T4 to T3, and decrease the amount of T3 being turned back into T4. Some vitamins and nutrients encourage the production of hormones. See Chapter Nine for a program of supplements designed for thyroid health.

Jennifer

Jennifer came to me with Hashimoto's disease—and joint pain, as well as a number of other complaints. As with all of my patients with autoimmune disorders, I looked for the underlying cause. What was sending her immune system into red alert? I suspected overexposure to heavy metals or other toxins, or perhaps a chronic infection that had evaded diagnosis. In my practice, the preponderance of patients with autoimmune illnesses of any kind, and knee pain to go along with it, get relief from their knee pain when the immune problem is ferreted out and treated.

Eventually I discovered Jennifer had a parasitic infection, which we were able to clear up with a combination of prescription antibiotics, herbs, and nutritional support. Once the infection cleared, not only did her thyroid levels normalize but her joint pain and other symptoms vanished as well.

It would seem like a remarkable recovery if not for the fact that I see cases like this probably every week. What was notable to me was this: Jennifer used a mail-order pharmacy to order medications and process her lab tests. One day she got a call from a nurse practitioner at the lab—which was itself a forward thinking medical establishment, I might add—who had noticed her lab tests for thyroid antibodies had been showing steadily decreasing levels. The nurse wanted to know how on earth Jennifer had managed that since she herself had been diagnosed with Hashimoto's and had always been told that her problem could only be controlled and that her antibodies would be present forever.

Causes of Hormonal Imbalance

Menopause and perimenopause may be the most obvious causes of hormonal imbalance and knee pain, but there are several other very common scenarios you should be aware of as well.

Insulin resistance

Insulin resistance, which sixty to eighty million Americans already have, and the number keeps growing, can create hormonal imbalances that will affect your knees. In insulin resistance, the cells are unable to use insulin (a hormone) to handle sugar and simple carbohydrate metabolism. In the extreme, this is type 2 diabetes.

Insulin resistance leads to abnormal glycemic control, and thus sugar levels that can be either too high or too low. You might also hear the term "hypoglycemia." There are essentially two kinds of hypoglycemia, the first of which is a full-blown disease resulting in too much insulin, as from an insulin-secreting tumor. That is technically the disease hypoglycemia. More often what we are talking about when we say hypoglycemia is what is more properly known as "functional reactive hypoglycemia," and features fierce cravings for carbs, an inability to lose weight and fatigue after a meal. The better name for that is insulin resistance. Your insulin levels are actually high because your body is insensitive to it—is unable to use it—and so sugar doesn't get into the cells, and the body keeps producing more insulin to try to do the job.

Women with insulin resistance already have increased inflammatory reactions, like those associated with rapidly changing estrogen levels.

But insulin resistance also contributes directly to hormonal imbalance by increasing testosterone, increasing estrogen, and eliminating or reducing the natural and crucial cyclical peaks of estrogen.

If you have insulin resistance, you must correct it before you can balance your hormones properly. Your glucose-to-insulin ratio (determined by a blood test) should be equal to or less than 9 to 1. Please note that that is probably *not* the figure your doctor will give you. Officially, insulin is considered normal at 12 or 14 (when you've been fasting), and mainstream medicine doesn't consider it dangerous until it hits the 15 to 20 range. However, I firmly believe even an 8 or 9 should serve as a warning sign. In addition, patients have increased and decreased blood sugar levels during the day, depending on their diet and lifestyle. It is not unusual to have "normal" insulin levels and be, in fact, insulin resistant, so I'd put more stock in your symptoms than your lab results.

Insulin resistance can also cause hyperglycemia (the best example being type 2 diabetes) as well as hypoglycemia, though the latter is more common early on in the process. As time goes on, your sugar levels will vary from too low to too high—not high enough to diagnose diabetes but higher than we would like to see, say in the mid or high nineties—and later still you might actually develop diabetes, at which point your sugar will usually or always be too high. Whether your sugar is high or low as a result of insulin resistance, the same inappropriate hormone conversions can result.

PMS

The unpleasant symptoms of PMS are caused by hormonal imbalances, and cyclical hormone fluctuation can cause the same problems as longer term trends, such as estrogen dominance or progesterone deficiency. Many of my patients report that their knee pain comes and goes in concert with their menstrual cycle. In some women with PMS, as their estrogen-to-progesterone ratio fluctuates and they become progesterone deficient—especially those with insulin resistance or carbohydrate intolerance—or when they are under chronic stress, their hormone levels shift enough to put them into a hypoglycemic state. The combination of dropping progesterone and low sugar will stimulate adrenaline release. When the body has more adrenaline than it can deal with, the excess tends to find its way into the synovial fluid and tissue surrounding the joints—creating inflammation and knee pain.

Research shows that women who are insulin resistant tend to be deficient in progesterone premenstrually, and the resulting adrenaline release creates those nervous, anxious, moody side effects (and could cause knee pain as well). That's why when you are PMS-ing, you crave carbs and unleash all your bad habits. It's the insulin resistance manifesting, with progesterone deficiency as the precipitating factor. Fortunately, taking progesterone solves the problem. (Again, you must take care of insulin resistance first. In fact, before you use over-the-counter hormones of any type, you must know that you are otherwise healthy and that they are appropriate for you.) Patients who are hypoglycemic—who have functional reactive hypoglycemia—and have progesterone deficiency will get the same adrenaline release symptoms.

Because insulin resistance is a process that develops slowly over time, if you seem prone to insulin resistance (i.e., obesity or diabetes runs in your family) but don't yet show it on lab tests, and you are low in progesterone, you should start taking measures to be sure your progesterone levels remain normal and in good balance with your estrogen, to prevent the full blossoming of the resistance.

Stress

One of the effects of stress in your body—stress of any kind, from any cause—is to alter the normal conversion of one hormone into another, which can result in the kind of hormonal imbalances we've been discussing in this chapter.

In addition, stress produces adrenaline, which as I've said before has an affinity for the synovial fluid within the joints, including the knee. If you do not use that adrenaline productively, for instance by exercising, the excess will be stored in and attach to the membranes in the joint, decreasing blood flow and creating an irritation and possibly an inflammation. (See also Chapter Seven on stress.)

In today's world, however, our stresses tend to stick around for months or even years. Our adrenaline never gets a chance to let up. But still our body considers it a matter of survival (though, if we really stop to think about it, a cranky boss and too many soccer league obligations are not actually life-or-death situations). The body therefore deems meeting the demands of stress to be much more important than having sex, or successfully reproducing—or living without knee pain—and is ready, willing and able to throw over the controls for all those things in the interest of pumping out the adrenaline (during the initial stress) and DHEA or cortisol (over the long haul, when the stress becomes chronic) it thinks you need. It does so at whatever cost, including cannibalizing sex hormones to reconvert them into stress hormones, and you can just imagine what kind of uproar that can create in your body.

Because long-term stress means an increase in cortisol levels, your thyroid is at risk, too: Increasing cortisol creates an increase in reverse T3. Reverse T3 inhibits its namesake thyroid hormone—if T3 is the gas pedal, reverse T3 is the brake. So an increase in reverse T3 decreases the body's available level of normal T3, and leads to all the symptoms of hypothyroidism (see box at the end of this chapter), including weak muscles and joint pain. But your thyroid levels will still test out normally (at mainstream labs, anyway). That's because reverse T3 is structurally similar enough (a mirror image, actually) to T3 to hook up to your body's T3 receptors, but faces the wrong direction so the receptors won't pick it up. Effectively, reverse T3 physically blocks the body from using T3. So you'll have what should be enough T3 in your blood, making the tests come out normal, but your cells will have a definite deficiency of T3 and all the hypothyroid symptoms that go along with that.

Increased cortisol is bad for you, just like taking the drug cortisone for a long time is bad for you. But long-term stress eventually results in *low* cortisol levels—which is *very* bad. With cortisol too low, you can't heal or fight pain or put out inflammation—you are too busy trying to survive, and all the nutrients you take in are pressed into service that way. If you don't survive, who cares if your knee hurts?

The "saber-toothed tiger" theory of stress holds that we learned our stress response way back in the days when we might have met one of those predators face to face. When that happened, adrenaline surged in the "fight or flight" response, helping us defend our survival or get to safety. When the immediate danger passed and we rested, the stress hormones receded.

And, when the stress doesn't go away, adrenaline alone can't keep up, and the body also produces DHEA and cortisol. You'll be converting estrogen and testosterone that should have important business elsewhere into DHEA and cortisol, furthering hormone-balance chaos. Your levels of DHEA and cortisol may be alternatively too high and too low when stress is more or less continuous and your body produces and devours them as fast as it can. Eventually, your levels will both be too low and you have no reserve. This is when you "crash."

Pain—like knee pain—may result in your body producing still more cortisol to reduce the inflammation. Getting too much cortisol from your body can have the same effects as taking a prescription for cortisol over the long run: fluid and electrolyte abnormalities, osteo- porosis and even spontaneous fractures, and, to make it a source of knee pain, muscle weakness and wasting. High levels of DHEA can result in abnormal levels of testosterone, estrogen, and other hormones affected by this chain reaction.

Poor nutrition

Poor nutrition can also throw off the balance of your hormones. Your body needs nutrients in order to manufacture the hormones. You may remember that the basic structure of hormones is composed of choles- terol. The type of cholesterol you produce is dependent not on the cho- lesterol in your diet, which despite the hype actually has little bearing on the situation, but on the type of fats you provide your body with. You need plenty of good fats, healthy unsaturated fats, such as omega- 3 and omega-6 and other essential fatty acids found in fish, seeds and nuts. (See Chapter Five for more on getting healthy fats into your diet and avoiding unhealthy ones, and Chapter Nine for information about essential fatty acid supplements.) Some high quality saturated fats are also helpful.

Excessive exercise

Excessive exercise alters the balance of hormones as well, the classic (though extreme) example being the runner who trains so much, and gets her body fat so low, that her body can't produce normal levels of sex hormones and she stops menstruating. Stressful exercise (too much, too long, too hard) increases stress hormones and decreases sex hormones. Exercise should be healing, not hurting. How much exercise is too much will be different for everyone, but in general, keep in mind that you should never be more than just a little fatigued by it, and that no one should exercise for hours every day, exercise all the same muscles every day, or exercise to the point of exhaustion.

You could be overexercising to the detriment of your hormones long before your menstrual cycle would stop. At the outset, your body would compensate for the excessive demands you were placing on it; but it couldn't keep that up indefinitely, and your hormones would be abnormal for a long time before your periods would actually stop. You would have symptoms of hormone imbalance as described in the boxes at the end of this chapter. So if you recognize yourself in one of them, you should take a look at your exercise habits, among other things.

Synthetic or foreign hormones

Estrogen (as well as every other hormone) comes in many different forms, and each form is broken down and used by the body in a distinct way. Natural hormones, such as natural estriol (an estrogen), for example, is used immediately in the body and leaves behind no debris. Synthetic hormones, which are not biologically identical to what your body produces even if they go by the same general name, break down less cleanly, requiring additional detoxification by the liver and still leaving behind debris. That debris can be carcinogenic and/or oxidative—and it can cause, among many other things, inflammation in the joints.

Standard hormone replacement therapy (HRT) is synthetic or, in the case of the most commonly prescribed estrogen, "natural" (from horse urine) but foreign to the human body. (It is possible, and just as easy, to get all-natural hormone replacement, however.) Hormonal birth control uses synthetic hormones as well. We are also exposed to foreign hormones from contaminated food and plastics, as we've discussed.

Rebalancing Hormones

Balancing your hormones will lessen the release of inflammatory agents, relieving your knee pain. You shouldn't escape your monthly cycle, and you can't turn back the clock, but in most cases proper diet, supplements, stress-reduction techniques and occasionally (natural) supplemental hormones almost always do the trick.

The first thing to do is to establish what your hormone levels are and see if they are, in fact, out of balance. Your doctor can check via a blood test. Some labs only offer basic hormone tests, while others allow more complete analysis of the metabolism of hormones. Saliva tests are a noninvasive alternative, and make it easy to check at various times of the day and on various days of the menstrual cycle if that is relevant. But be warned that only a limited number of practitioners use them—although why they aren't more widely used mystifies me. In Europe urine tests are widely used, but the large commercial labs in this country don't seem to do them, and again I am baffled as to why this extremely accurate, well-studied method is overlooked (except by researchers and specialty labs, who do use them!).

If all you have available to you are blood tests, you should get an early morning blood draw after you've fasted overnight, somewhere between days nineteen and twenty-five of your menstrual cycle, and again on a day when you have PMS or other types of recurrent symptoms. That way you can compare the results against a known standard as well as against each other, to see what hormone levels might be related to your symptoms.

There are also tests that will reveal what you are metabolizing your estrogen into, giving you the ability to zero in on where in the cascade of hormones you are going off balance—and so know where and how to correct it. You have several types of estrogen, some safer than others, circulating in your body at all times. Every cell in your body has receptors for estrogen. Which types of estrogen you have available to those receptors—which types of estrogen your body actually gets to put into use—dictates how your cells will react and function. Your body breaks down estrogen into many different forms (metabolites), and by testing for specific metabolites you can see how much of which types of estrogen your body is using. You can surmise how much of the safest types of estrogen you have, and what you need to do to increase them if necessary.

There have been plenty of great peer-reviewed research articles published about this over the last few years, but no regular labs do the testing yet since so very few doctors order it. There are high-quality labs that specialize in functional medicine that *do* do the test, however, and if your regular doctor isn't familiar with it, it may well be worth it to seek out a more naturally oriented health-care provider to help you get this crucial information about your body. It's very important for several reasons, not the least of which is that some hormonal metabolites are more strongly correlated with breast cancer and other problems. If the results indicate that your body is likely burdened with a lot of debris, you can change the type of estrogen you are taking (if indeed you are taking estrogen), or you can use nutritional supplements and good dietary practices to normalize your estrogen metabolism. Even in menopause, you still have to make sure the hormones your body is producing stay in balance with each other. When they do not, simply taking hormones without determining why your body is not functioning at its best runs you the risk of creating an even worse imbalance (even if some hormone levels seem to improve)—and certainly doesn't address the cause of the imbalance. You should be able to get your body to produce fewer undesirable hormones and more desirable ones within

STEROID HORMONE METABOLISM

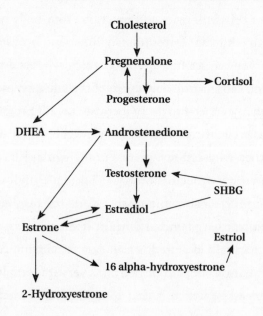

only two months with the appropriate dietary changes and nutritional (*not* hormonal) supplements.

Once you know where you stand with your hormones, rebalancing them is a matter of proper nutrition (as described in Chapters Five and Nine), exercise (Chapters Six and Ten), stress reduction (Chapter Seven) and possibly supplementary hormones. If you do take hormones, the specific types and dosages must be tailored to your particular situation. One or two standard variations in dosage will never be able to meet everyone's individual needs, although that seems to be mainstream medicine's assumption. Not everyone needs to take hormones to stabilize the levels in their bodies, and not everyone who does decide to use hormones needs estradiol or progesterone. And I believe no one needs progestins, although they are found in the world's most commonly prescribed "progesterone" (a misnomer—they are really progestins, which are similar in some ways but definitely not the same as what your body manufactures or uses).

Everyone who does use hormones should investigate *natural* forms. What research into supplemental hormones and knee pain exists shows a benefit from standard hormone replacement therapy—meaning synthetic hormones. My experience with my patients is that they get even better results with fewer or no side effects when they use all-natural hormones because they are structurally identical to what your body makes. Consider this: While estrogen and testosterone, which obviously have dramatically different effects on the body, differ only by about one hydrogen ion (as mentioned previously), natural and synthetic estrogen or progesterone differ by at least forty or fifty structures and can be thirty to fifty times stronger than your body's natural hormones! Just imagine how distinct their impacts can be. Furthermore, for the body to use the synthetic hormones, it must break them down into a chemical it recognizes, and doing so frequently leaves behind a great deal of debris your body must then detoxify and/or excrete if it can. When you can't do it well, you experience side effects, if not diseases.

When you think about it, these side effects are predictable. We know a certain percentage of people will experience these side effects every time they use any drug that is metabolized the same way. We also know that in this population of genetically sensitive people, everyone will experience these predictable effects. That means you will most likely react (both positively and negatively) the way your mother did.

I3C (indole-3-carbonol) or DIM (diindolylmethane), both of which are available at your local health-food store, change the way your body metabolizes the estrogen you take and/or the estrogen your body produces, resulting in the availability of safer estrogens for your body's use. DIM has a stronger, more focused action (to the point that it can occasionally be too strong for someone) while I3C, for which there is more research, has a broader range. DIM is a product of broken-down I3C, and the two work in essentially the same way. Most products now contain both.

Flax seed, soy, and kudzu can also help by acting as adaptogenic herbs that can balance estrogen levels and help in estrogen metabolism. (For more information, see Chapters Five and Nine.)

Diet and supplements help improve thyroid function as well. Vitamins A and D are prohormones that stimulate the thyroid as well as improve immune function. Insulin-stabilizing nutrients such as essential fatty acids (EFAs), chromium and cadmium decrease reverse T3, as do herbs known as guggals, the herb *Withania somnifera* (also known as ashwagandha), and conjugated linoleic acid. Selenium, zinc, guggals and *Withania somnifera* also increase T3 levels. You can help your body convert T4 to T3 with guggals (which also decrease LDL cholesterol by improving mitochondrial function), selenium and zinc. With the right diet and nutritional supplements, you can make sure normal T3 is available in your body at normal levels.

Several supplements increase not only your thyroid hormone levels but also your body's sensitivity to thyroid hormones (via increasing thyroid hormone receptor activity). They include the essential fatty acids DHA, EPA and CLA; carnosic acid (found in rosemary) as well as vitamins A and D.

Gina

Gina was only in her mid-thirties but already having menopausal symptoms, including irregular periods, hot flashes, changes in breast tissue, fatigue, digestive problems, insomnia or fitful sleep, low energy, dry skin—and joint pain. Her knees were swollen, stiff and painful. She lived with a lot of stress in her life, both physical and emotional. She was quick to sacrifice to make sure the needs of those around her were met. Her diet wasn't horrible, but she was always eating on the run, which is never a recipe for well-balanced nutrition. She exercised regularly (and aggressively), but it sapped rather than replenished her energy, and her muscles always hurt afterward. It would take days for her to recover, and since she didn't wait days before working out again, the exercise itself was stressful rather than healing.

A physical and history didn't find any particular smoking gun. But her thyroid hormones were just slightly low, and saliva tests done as many as six times a day revealed her stress hormones to be out of whack, with cortisol too high at some times of day and too low at others, and DHEA consistently too low. Her sex hormones too were a little off, with estrogen and progesterone each at normal levels—but imbalanced in relationship to each other. Her testosterone was also low. Her body was no doubt converting sex hormones into DHEA trying to cope with the demands of stress, but that can only be a stopgap measure. The stress was so constant that DHEA levels were finally low despite the backward conversions, and the reproductive hormones were therefore off too—and so Gina's menopausal symptoms were born. And her knees began to ache.

I had a custom hormone replacement cream formulated for Gina, using only natural hormones structurally identical to what the body itself produces. I don't like to give a lot of hormones at once, as it is hard to regulate and balance them. I decide on the one or two prime suspects, and monitor the others right along with them. Most times, with the correct raw materials on hand in adequate amounts, the hormones will balance themselves. For Gina, the most important hormones in her cream were DHEA and testosterone.

She called within a week to thank me for this "magic." She simply felt much better. Her energy level was up, and her general sense of well-being restored. She was sleeping at night, thinking clearly, and no longer having hot flashes. I don't want to give all the credit to the cream—along with using natural hormones, Gina modified her exercise program, cleaned up her diet and starting taking a program of supplements. As her hormones started to properly align themselves, her thyroid levels normalized too. I wasn't too surprised—it wasn't that the thyroid gland wasn't producing suitable stuff, it was that the cells couldn't use what was being made because of adrenal malfunction. And, finally, her knees stopped hurting.

Suffice it to say that this is a very complicated emerging area of medicine, and an entire book could be devoted to how to keep your hormones in balance. Everyone should check to be sure they are in fact in balance, and take steps to get in balance if they are not. The best way to do this is to work with a holistic doctor and/or nutritionist or other professional to find a natural way to rebalance your hormones, reserving taking hormones, even natural hormones, as a last resort. Try to eliminate the need for additional hormones rather than temporarily supplying what your body should be able to manage on its own, which only covers over your problem without solving it. But if you do need hormones, then you should definitely go the extra mile to find natural ones that are chemically the same as what your body makes and uses.

You can start on your own by perusing the boxes at the end of this chapter to see if any of those collections of symptoms sounds all too familiar. That will give you a suspected culprit to focus on. Get the relevant blood, urine or saliva tests. If you have symptoms, do not accept an answer of "everything's normal." If your regular doctor interprets your tests that way, you may need to seek out a holistic practitioner with a subtler understanding of hormones. Everything is not normal if you do not feel in optimal health. You may not have a disease, but as long as you have dis-ease, something is not functioning well and you should get to the bottom of it. It may be the solution to your knee pain (as well as to so much more).

SYMPTOMS OF ESTROGEN DEFICIENCY

- Vaginal dryness
- Night sweats
- Bladder infections
- Incontinence
- Sleep disturbance
- Painful intercourse
- Memory problems
- Hot flashes
- Lethargic depression/ tearful depression
- Foggy thinking
- Bone loss
- Palpitations

SYMPTOMS OF EXCESS ESTROGEN

- Foggy thinking
- Weepiness
- Gallbladder problems
- Fibrocystic breast
- Water retention around your hips
- Puffiness and bloating
- Rapid weight gain around your hips
- Breast tenderness
- Mood swings (PMS)
- Heavy bleeding
- Anxiety
- Depression
- Irritability
- Migraines
- Cervical dysplasia (abnormal pap smear)
- Fibroids
- Insomnia
- Red flush on face

SYMPTOMS OF CORTISOL DEFICIENCY

- Debilitating fatigue
- Sugar craving
- Unstable blood sugar
- Foggy thinking
- Low blood pressure
- Thin and/or dry skin
- Intolerance to exercise
- Allergies
- Chemical sensitivity
- Stress
- Brown spots on face
- Cold body temperature
- Palpitations
- Aches and pains

SYMPTOMS OF EXCESS CORTISOL

- Sleep disturbance
- Fatigue
- Depression
- Thinning skin
- Bone loss
- Decreased muscle mass

SYMPTOMS OF PROGESTERONE DEFICIENCY

- PMS
- Insomnia
- Early miscarriage
- Vaginal dryness
- Unexplained weight gain
- Foggy thinking
- Water retention
- Early bone loss
- Memory lapses
- Hot flashes
- Incontinence
- Anxiety
- Heart palpitations
- Painful and/or lumpy breasts
- Tearfulness
- Cyclical headaches
- Infertility

SYMPTOMS OF EXCESS PROGESTERONE

- Breast swelling/tenderness
- Decreased libido
- Mild depression
- Yeast infection

SYMPTOMS OF ESTROGEN DOMINANCE

- Symptoms of excess estrogen AND deficient progesterone

SYMPTOMS OF TESTOSTERONE DEFICIENCY

- Decreased libido
- Fatigue
- Depression
- Sleep disturbance
- Bone loss
- Decreased muscle mass
- Vaginal dryness
- Foggy thinking
- Aches and pains
- Memory lapses
- Incontinence
- Thinning skin

SYMPTOMS OF EXCESS TESTOSTERONE

- Acne
- Polycystic ovary syndrome (POCS)
- Excessive hair on face and arms
- Ovarian cysts
- Hypoglycemia or unstable blood sugar
- Mid-cycle pain
- Infertility

SYMPTOMS OF PARASITES

- Gas
- Bloating
- Reflux
- Constipation
- Diarrhea
- Fatigue
- Malnutrition
- History of food poisoning or dysentery
- Unexplained chronic illness

SYMPTOMS OF LOW THYROID

- Low body temperature
- Cold hands and feet
- Unexplained weight gain/ inability to lose weight
- Dry skin
- Fatigue

- Constipation
- Stiff or aching joints
- Hair loss
- Soft or brittle fingernails
- High cholesterol

SYMPTOMS OF HIGH THYROID

- Increased blood pressure
- Flushing from overeating
- Profuse perspiration
- Nervousness
- Sleeplessness
- Diarrhea
- Rapid heartbeat

5

Nourish Your Knees

You might be eating your way right into joint pain. It might be a direct connection (putting too much stress on the knees by gaining weight), or it might be more subtle but just as damaging (starting a chain reaction that leads to inflammation in the knee by eating inflammation-producing foods and/or not eating sufficiently nutritious foods). Fortunately, you can also eat to heal and restore your knees, relieving your knee pain. This chapter shows you how, with guidance on what to eat—on both the macro and micro levels—to maintain a healthy weight as well as provide your knees with the nutrients they need to stay supple.

Lose Weight

To begin with, being overweight greatly increases your risk of developing knee pain. Simply put, it increases the load the knees have to cope with, causing excessive strain. Overweight women have twice the risk of developing knee pain as compared to women of a healthy weight. It doesn't take a whole lot of excess weight for this effect to kick in. Losing even ten pounds can decrease your pain, or your risk of pain. (Though losing another ten pounds will be more helpful, and so on, until you reach an all-around healthy weight.)

Being overweight is well established as a risk factor specifically for osteoarthritis. It probably makes more difference in whether or not you develop OA than in how the condition progresses once you have it. The effect is most noticeable in the ten or so years preceding menopause—which holds even when you control for other relevant factors, such as use of supplemental estrogen, height, smoking and access to health-care providers. Studies show that women who have osteoarthritis weigh about 15 percent more than women who don't.

So watching what you eat—not just how much you eat, but what it consists of—in the interest of maintaining a stable, healthy weight may be your single best bet to prevent and reverse knee pain. It is definitely not just a matter of how many calories you consume. (You'll also need exercise, of course; see Chapters Six and Ten.) You should also make sure you have an honest assessment of your weight: A Gallup poll shows that while more than half of all Americans are, in point of fact, overweight, just 40 percent say they are overweight. That bit of denial may seem harmless, but it isn't if it keeps you from hearing the warning bells that are going off about your health, including your knees. Your knees are realists and are definitely not influenced by your denial.

Build Up Cartilage

The knee-nutrition connection goes deeper than weight. Including the right raw materials in your diet allows your body to create and maintain the cartilage, ligament, tendon, bone and muscle that are critical to joint health. You need, in particular, plenty of vitamins C and E, B vitamins, calcium, magnesium, zinc, copper, manganese, molybdenum, boron, L-lysine, bromelain, essential fatty acids, and L-proline. And you will get all or most of these necessary nutrients if you eat a variety of foods, including fruit (especially berries), vegetables (especially cruciferous and green leafy), vegetable oils, nuts, whole grains, beans and legumes, meats, eggs and cold-water fish. If for whatever reason you can't eat enough of the food you need, you can always add supplements to make up the difference. You'll also benefit from glucosamine and chondroitin, and the herbs hawthorn and horsetail, though getting those will require supplements. (Chapter Nine will cover supplements.)

Cool Inflammation

If your body does not have all the nutrients it needs, you cannot keep up with all the demands you make on your body. Plus, when the demands you make create oxidation and free radicals as well as waste products that cause inflammation, then you won't be able to handle that either: a double whammy. That inflammation can occur anywhere in your body, although the knee is a very popular spot. Lack of nutrients also results in the formation of poorer quality structures such as bone and cartilage.

Inflammation is a normal bodily process. It is how the body repairs tissue damage and protects against infection. The body releases prostaglandins, which are inflammatory (as well as healing), and, if all goes well, stops releasing them when the tissue heals. When inflammation is chronic, as with arthritis, the process runs wild.

The quality of the nutrients in your diet—particularly healthful fatty acids and antioxidants—greatly influence the action of prostaglandins—hormones that, among other things, moderate inflammation. Prostaglandins' cousins, leukotrienes—fat components that also moderate inflammation as well as control swelling and stimulate the release of prostaglandins—likewise feel the effects of poor nutrition.

Including plenty of high-quality essential fatty acids (EFAs) in your diet is one of the simplest and best ways to fight excess inflammation. Fats are what you manufacture all of your sex and stress hormones from. They are also beneficial for the heart, brain, nervous system and more. So despite the "low-fat" brainwashing we've all been subject to, essential fatty acids—and lots of them—are all-around good for you. Choose high-quality EFAs, which include unsaturated, monounsaturated and polyunsaturated fats; when you hear about "omega-3s" and "omega-6s," what's being referred to are EFAs. Fish, nuts, seeds and some grains, and eggs are the best sources, and we'll get into more specifics on that a little later in this chapter. Fruits are good too, as they contain a lot of bioflavonoids and other anti-inflammatory substances, so you should eat a variety of them. Citrus fruits, tomatoes, plums and berries in an array of colors are especially helpful. Cruciferous vegetables such as broccoli, cauliflower, brussels sprouts, cabbage and kale are also beneficial, as are beans and legumes, onions, rhubarb, parsley, ginger, turmeric, cayenne and green tea. Avocados contain healthy fats and oils, which are of prime importance in an anti-inflammatory diet.

Eat Right for . . . Everything

Besides nourishing your knees, fighting inflammation and stabilizing weight, the eating plan laid out in this chapter will also help balance your hormones (see Chapter Four for more on the importance of that). On top of that, it is what your whole body needs anyway to be healthy, no matter what particular perspective you're starting from—it's good for your heart, your bones, your brain . . . you name it.

In fact, one of the most beneficial effects of this way of eating is to stave off Syndrome X, also known as the metabolic syndrome or the insulin resistance syndrome, a cluster of disorders including high blood sugars (and in the extreme, type 2 diabetes), high blood pressure, high LDL cholesterol (the "bad" one), low HDL cholesterol (the "good" one), elevated triglycerides, obesity, high uric acid, heart disease, stroke and more. Hormone-linked problems, such as irregular menstrual cycles and polycystic ovary syndrome, can also be part of Syndrome X. At least one-quarter of Americans have Syndrome X—and the increased risk of heart attack, stroke and organ damage that comes with it—and that figure is steadily growing.

While the exact disorders that show up in any individual case of Syndrome X vary, what is universal is the way the cells of the body lose their sensitivity to insulin, which is why this condition is also known as insulin resistance. Insulin works to control blood sugar levels, and move sugar from the blood into the cells of the muscles, liver, brain and so on, for your body to burn as fuel. When your body isn't responding to insulin, you can't properly use glucose for energy. Insulin also regulates how your body metabolizes, packages and stores fat to meet your energy requirements.

Actually, the better name for this condition, and one that is starting to come into favor, is "metabolic syndrome." Whatever you call it, the bottom line is that it is a pro-inflammatory metabolism, and knee pain will often pop up on the list of connected symptoms.

Insulin resistance has reached epidemic proportions in this country, and is wreaking havoc with a great many people's health. The backbone of the eating plan I recommend here is basically designed to prevent and reverse it. I've then tailored it to keeping knees healthy. You'll not only be able to stabilize at a healthy weight (without counting calories)—taking a lot of the pressure off your joints in the process—but also deal with a host of chronic and potentially deadly conditions. As a bonus (if all this wasn't enough already), you'll feel less foggy and much more energetic when you switch over to eating this way.

When you eat carbohydrates, especially simple carbohydrates, which the body handles the same way as sugar, they are rapidly absorbed into the bloodstream, dramatically raising blood sugar levels and triggering the release of insulin. This is the normal response of the body. When you overeat simple carbohydrates over a long period of time, you change your metabolism from what we accept as "normal" to your *new* normal of a carbohydrate-based metabolism, and this potentiates the process of insulin resistance. When you do this over the long run, for many if not most or all of us, it results in a decreasing sensitivity to insulin. Since your insulin isn't working efficiently, your body responds by producing more insulin. The increased insulin overprocesses the sugar, and within a few hours, your blood sugar is even lower than it was before you ate. Now, your body feels like it is out of fuel; you feel hungry, tired and crave sugar and other carbohydrates—starting the cycle all over again. This goes for everyone, but when you are insulin resistant, the cycle is even more vicious. On top of it, the more you weigh, the more insulin your pancreas will release, and the more likely you are to develop insulin resistance—making you even more likely to gain weight!

The typical person with this syndrome is thin as a child, and can eat everything and anything, especially junk food and carbs, and not gain weight as their parents did. Then "all of a sudden," when they hit their forties, they start to gain weight, change shape, and develop the metabolic changes associated with long-term insulin resistance.

Supplements for Syndrome X

To prevent or reverse Syndrome X (aka metabolic syndrome, or insulin resistance syndrome), you need to get plenty of insulin-balancing nutrients. (You'll find more information on many of these supplements in Chapter Nine). These nutrients in particular can be beneficial in dealing with Syndrome X:

- Acetyl L-carnitine
- Alpha lipoic acid
- Cadmium (stabilizes insulin)
- Chromium (stabilizes insulin)
- Conjugated linoleic acid (CLA)
- L-arginine
- L-carnitine
- Magnesium
- Manganese
- Omega-3s
- Omega-6s
- Selenium
- Vanadium
- Vanadyl sulfate
- Vitamin C
- Vitamin D
- Vitamin E
- Zinc

Herbs can also be beneficial, including:

- Bay leaves
- Bitter melon
- Cinnamon
- Cloves
- Colosolic acid
- Coriander
- Fenugreek (reduces blood sugar)
- Garlic (regulates cholesterol, supports blood vessels, treats diabetes)
- Green and black tea
- Gymnema sylvestre (balances blood sugar)
- Holy basil
- Nopal
- Salvia
- Silymarin (milk thistle) (detoxifies liver)
- Stevia

You could add just about any culinary herb or spice to this list, to the degree that they replace salt in your diet. They'll be helping.

Not everyone with Syndrome X will need or benefit from everything on this list. For instance, the more you exercise, the less carnitine, vitamin A and lipoic acid you will need. The more carbs you eat, the more chromium, vanadyl sulfate and gymnema sylvestre you will need.

Look for combination products with a good range of these nutrients. See Chapter Nine for more information on using supplements.

Eat Fat

Let me warn you now that this eating plan will not look very much like the famous food pyramid the government recommends. In a way it turns the food pyramid upside down, advising you to make sure you get *enough* fat in your diet. Don't expect Atkins style "eat all the meat and cheese you want" advice either, though. One of the best studies we have of nutrition and health—in which researchers at the Harvard School of Public Health have followed three hundred thousand people over the long haul—shows that the low-fat mantra is, at best, misguided and has most likely spurred the dramatic increase in obesity and, I believe, insulin resistance in this country. (The American Diabetic Association, the American Medical Association and other widely respected institutions concur with these findings.) If you've tried to lose weight by cutting out fat and relying on carbs instead, you (like almost everybody else) already know how often that fails—and it's been proven to do so in official studies as well as in everyday life.

In the two decades since the unveiling of the food pyramid ushered in the low-fat era, Americans have only gotten fatter—and sicker, as diabetes, heart disease and hypertension are more common now than ever. Although we're eating less fat, that's not solving our national cholesterol problem or the heart disease it is tied to. In fact, it is apparently making it worse: The rate of heart disease has gone up, and the risk of heart disease has gone up even more sharply. Among other things, this is a reminder that it is more than high cholesterol levels that cause heart disease. Most experts agree that our old friend inflammation is the real culprit—and cholesterol is actually an anti-inflammatory agent. In most people the inflammation that causes coronary artery disease is an immune response to some chronic battle they are waging—against infection, for example, or a toxin from the environment, a food they are sensitive to, or insulin resistance.

For up to 40 percent of Americans, low-fat diets actually cause weight gain, and for about 30 percent they actually *increase* the risk of heart disease. That's because we're eating more and more carbohydrates. Each of us downs thirty more pounds of sweeteners per year than we did twenty years ago, and about sixty more pounds of grains (most in the form of simple, processed carbs). We now average four hundred more calories each and every day than before the advent of the low-fat food pyramid! The lack of exercise, right down to the use of remote controls for the television, only makes it worse.

The problem with the low-fat diet isn't just the lack of fat per se, but also the quality of the fats, and the overreliance on carbohydrates. Americans have a diet very high in saturated and trans-fatty acids. If you replaced all the fat and protein you cut out with vegetables, you'd probably stay trim. But the human body was never designed to function like this. Let me give you just two examples of the importance of and need for fat. Earlier in this chapter I told you that all your sex and stress hormones are manufactured from fat. I'd also like to point out that 60 percent of the material in the brain that isn't water is fat—all of which comes from your diet. The membranes around each and every cell, which control all the information going into and out of that cell, are made of fat.

And, as hunter/gatherers, we never had much in the way of simple carbs until we invented agriculture about ten thousand years ago, a mere blip of time in the evolutionary sense. The human diet always consisted of free-range organic meats, plenty of organic fruits and vegetables and the unsaturated and saturated fats that come from high quality organic free-range sources. I am suggesting that we get back to this form of eating, which, after all, is what Mother Nature intended for us.

More often than not, we try to be healthy by cutting the fats in our diets, only to replace them with processed carbohydrates. Too often, our "healthy" diets look something like this: a huge fat-free muffin for breakfast, a plain bagel and a sweetened fat-free yogurt for lunch and a big bowl of pasta for dinner. But there is little of nutritional value there, just on overload of simple carbs.

In addition to wreaking havoc on our insulin resistance, studies show that a diet high in simple carbohydrates also increases the risk of heart disease. By now we've all heard that high LDL cholesterol is associated with heart disease, but high triglyceride levels are at least as common in people with heart disease—and a diet high in carbohydrates will increase triglyceride levels in many people. And our low-fat diet is harming us in yet another way: When we do allow ourselves to eat fat, we tend to gorge on the (good-tasting) hydrogenated fats packed into processed foods (also generally filled with simple carbs) and miss out all together on the healthy EFAs and HDL-raising, LDL-lowering, anti-inflammatory unsaturated fats such as those found in olive oil, fish and nuts.

Slowly the medical world is realizing it has veered off course when it comes to recommendations about fat in the diet, and is leaving behind the low-fat/high-carb pyramid and recommending the inclusion of more (healthy, high-quality) fats, as the rapidly accumulating data supports. To help us on our way, we can look forward to the coming advent of food labels that indicate the presence of trans-fatty acids—any level of which is negative—and natural (healthier) cis-fatty acids, which are unsaturated essential fatty acids. (It is cis-fatty acids that transform into trans-fatty acids when heated or hydrogenated. Trans-fatty acids act basically like saturated fats, but their damage potential doesn't stop there: They also interfere with your body's use of essential fatty acids and are carcinogenic.)

What to Eat

The good news is that the right foods (balanced with exercise and nutritional supplements—see Chapters Ten and Nine) can prevent and treat knee pain. If you've eaten your way into it, you can eat your way back out. The main idea is to eat a variety of foods, keep your simple carbohydrates to a minimum, eat high-quality organic protein, include plenty of unsaturated fats and essential fatty acids, and eat tons of a large variety of vegetables and fruits. When you do eat saturated fats, they should be high-quality organic saturated fats.

Don't go hungry. Eat enough, and often enough, to be satisfied and to get the nutrients and fuel you need to function well and produce enough energy to do everything you need to do in a day. Don't overeat, of course, but there's no need to deprive yourself either. Eating this way (and taking the correct supplements) will change your metabolism, and eating "enough" will allow you to lose weight (or maintain a healthy weight) without counting calories. I feel strongly that it is better to measure the quality of what you eat than the quantity.

Your real goal here, however, isn't just to change your metabolism or lower your sugar levels or lower your cholesterol, or any specific indicator of that ilk, but to cure insulin resistance altogether and to be in balance nutritionally and metabolically. You *will* change your body's metabolic process so that blood sugar, cholesterol, fat storage, and energy production and usage—and let's not forget knee pain—will be improved. But that's all a shake-out of getting rid of insulin resistance. You'll need to do the strictest version of what is laid out here until you get past any cravings for carbohydrates. Then you'll be able to add some back in. Though it takes some of my patients up to four months, or as little as one day or one month to get to that point, I generally recommend two to three months.

While you are reading here about what to eat, keep in mind that, as detailed in Chapter Six, to change your body, make your metabolism more efficient, reach your ideal body weight, and take a load off your knees, you will also need to exercise. Aerobic exercise is particularly important.

Several components play into precisely how long you should follow this way of eating. In its most general form, it is meant to be a lifetime plan. And you'll need to start out strictly, as we've noted. From there, though, if you do more exercise and take supplements, you'll need to restrict your diet less or for a shorter time. If you eat well and exercise, you won't need as many supplements. And so on. Making best use of all three prongs will bring the fastest and most complete results. Continuing on the same path for a lifetime will ensure you the longest and healthiest life.

As for what you eat: Start with a focus on whole, unprocessed foods—foods the way Mother Nature made them, as natural and seasonally fresh as possible. Refined and processed foods are stripped of many nutrients. Eat free-range and organic foods to decrease foreign hormones, pesticides, toxins and many other pollutants that are found in our food chain. (Free-range means animals that not only are fed good food but also get regular exercise, and are therefore themselves healthier. Free-range isn't, however, always organic; both is best.)

Make your intake of carbohydrates moderate or low, but include substantial amounts of fiber, both soluble and insoluble. That fiber comes with complex carbohydrates, which are beneficial—it is simple carbs and sugars we have to eliminate. No sensible person should tell you to eliminate broccoli because of its carbs! Stick with complex carbohydrates—whole grains; vegetables; beans; legumes; raw, unprocessed nuts and seeds—which are high in fiber and rich in nutrients. Emphasize non-starchy vegetables in particular. Complex carbs take longer to be digested, so they have less of an impact on blood sugar and insulin levels. The body breaks down all carbs into sugar eventually, but the more complex the carbohydrate, the more steps in the process, and the fewer insulin surges will result. When I say whole grains, I mean *whole* whole grains; whole grain flours lose nutrients in processing and, in addition, are that much more quickly broken down into simple sugars. The more processed the grain is, the less nutritious.

Get five servings a day of foods high in soluble fibers, such as oat bran, old-fashioned (not instant or quick) oatmeal, barley, beans and legumes, and fruits. Flax seeds are an excellent source of fiber, as well as lignans (plant hormones) and omega-3s (linoleic acid and alpha linolenic acid). Have lots of whole grains—millet and buckwheat are great choices—followed by rye and wheat. Spelt, quinoa, and amaranth are also good, but should be used in moderation. Be careful if you are gluten sensitive; you'll have to avoid not only wheat but also rye, oats, barley and other mixed grains.

Skip sugar and other simple carbs, especially anything made out of white flour, which the body treats just like sugar. The one exception is fruit: Fruits are full of natural sugars, but they are otherwise rich and balanced nutritionally, and the fiber they contain slows the release of sugar into the bloodstream, more like complex carbohydrates. If you are having blood sugar problems you should limit grapes, bananas and pineapples, which are particularly hard on blood sugar levels, and cut out all dried fruit and fruit juice, which have concentrated sugars. Otherwise steer clear of sugar in any form, including fruit juice and fruit concentrates (which have no compensating fiber), maple syrup, honey, jams and jellies, and, that food processors' darling, high-fructose corn syrup. I recommend avoiding artificial sweeteners as well, because the body metabolizes them just as it does sugar. Read labels carefully; you'll be amazed where you will find sugar.

Sweets for the Sweet

If you must have a sweet taste, try using the herb stevia, which you can find in health food stores (¼ teaspoon = 2 tablespoons sugar). Or, try the nutritional supplements xylitol or FOS (fructo-oligo saccharides).

Potatoes turn into sugar very rapidly in the body, but sweet potatoes are actually okay because, on a chemical level, they don't interfere with your sugar levels as much. (Still, you should still probably hold it to three or four of them a week.) If you want bread, I'd suggest one slice a day of nine- or twelve-grain (making sure it is actually made with whole grains and whole grain flours—it should be chunky) or sprouted bread, but other than that you should cut way back on pasta, pancakes, bagels and all that stuff made with white and/or processed flour. Artichoke pasta is a good alternative. I learned from a patient of mine about Tinkyada brand pasta made from brown rice, or brown rice fortified with rice bran, which is delicious.

When you do indulge in carbs, don't eat them on their own—have a healthy source of protein or fat, such as olive oil or organic butter, at the same time to provide a bit of a cushion for what happens to your blood sugar. Fat and protein slow the absorption of sugar. And consider timing your intake of simple carbs for the first two hours after exercise, so your body can press them into immediate use.

As your weight (and blood sugar) stabilizes, you may well be able to tolerate more carbs without getting into the vicious cycle again. Most people should probably go two to three months sans carbs, or at least long enough for your cravings for them to stop, and you may be able to speed up the process by taking supplements. The stricter you are about what you eat, the faster you'll be able to ease up on those restrictions without plunging back into trouble.

Snacks are very important. They should be frequent enough—every two hours after breakfast and every three hours after lunch—to prevent your sugar levels from dropping far enough to force you to seek out the food you are trying to avoid. Eating healthy means *eating*, first and foremost. Don't go hungry, and never let yourself miss a meal.

You should have some protein at almost every meal and snack. Protein (as well as fat) slows digestion, and doesn't wreak so much havoc with blood sugar and insulin levels. It makes you feel sated, and keeps that feeling with you through to the next time you eat. Make your protein of the highest quality possible—whole; organic; free of hormones, pesticides and antibiotics. And make it free-range. Both you and the animals you eat should only ingest seasonally fresh, naturally whole foods. Organic, free-range filet mignon and fast-food chopped chuck burgers are both from cows, but they are far from nutritionally equal! It is a good idea to eat some non-starchy veggies along with any animal protein you have.

Because you should be limiting the amount of saturated fat you get, you shouldn't make meat your only source of protein. You'll get protein from beans, nuts, seeds and grains, but in addition you will want to make friends with the variety of soy products available today. If you aren't getting enough protein in your regular menu, you might want to use a soy amino-acid powder, as a drink or mixed in a hot or cold (whole grain) cereal. (You may want to keep your soy intake to no more than twenty-five to fifty grams, or about three ounces, a day if you have concerns about hormone balance [see Chapter Four].) You can use a whey protein powder the same way. Whey is a more neutral protein than soy and is a great choice for those who react to soy or need to limit soy.

The third major component of a healthy diet is fat: some high-quality saturated (animal) fats, mixed in with a variety of unsaturated fats. About 30 percent of your calories should come from a variety of healthy fats and oils: mono- and polyunsaturated, essential fatty acids (omega-3s and omega 6s), all of which you can get from food and/or supplements. Less than a third of that (that is, less than 10 percent of your calories overall) should come from saturated fat (which includes all animal fats). As with everything else, you'll do best with high-quality sources.

Don't avoid saturated fats altogether, however, because a combination and variety of many types of high-quality fats are important. Despite decades of anti-cholesterol, anti-fat hysteria, you actually need fat in your diet and in your life. DHEA, testosterone, estrogen and progesterone are made from cholesterol, as are cortisol, blood pressure hormones, and vitamin D, among other things. Without enough cholesterol you'll get a hormone imbalance, and the resultant inflammation and knee pain and all the other symptoms you don't want to experience.

Essential fatty acids are so called because your body needs them but does not make them; you could think of it being "essential" that you ingest them. There are two major types of EFAs that I think are important for your health: omega-3s and omega-6s, both of which decrease inflammation and the associated pain. The omega-6 DGLA, for example, is converted in the body into GLA (gamma linoleic acid), which is in turn transformed into prostaglandins, which your body uses to fight inflammation and pain. EFAs are also the raw material the body uses to make all the crucial sex hormones. All of the EFAs are converted into other EFAs and/or into prostaglandins and/or hormones, directly or indirectly. But not all of them can be used every way, so you need to get a variety of them.

Omega 3s include ALA (from flax seeds) and DHA (docasahexaenoic acid) and EPA, which are mostly found in deep-sea, cold-water fish, as well as in some northern plants (notably flax seeds and walnuts), some dark green plants (including algae), and soy (choose organic, non-genetically modified—the label should say non-GMO). (ALA and EPA are more important for the joints; DHA, while certainly good for you, is most beneficial for the brain.) Put a lot of deep-sea cold-water fish (see box on page 164) on your menus, the fattier the better. Free-range fish (not farm bred) have more omega-3s and fewer chemicals. You can also get omega-3 enriched eggs (with DHA or EPA) from chickens fed a particular kind of feed, and I'm here to tell you to forget your yolk phobia and enjoy up to as many as a dozen eggs a week, with the yellow stuff. (Even the traditional and conservative *Journal of the American Medical Association* recently published a study showing that eating as many as eight regular eggs a week did not raise cholesterol levels.)

Just the Flax

Flax seeds are an excellent source of fiber and lignans, as well as omega 3s. But you won't fully digest them if you eat them whole, so you'll miss out on a lot of the nutrients they have to offer. Buy whole flax seeds and grind some fresh every day or two in a coffee grinder. Sprinkle 1 to 2 tablespoons onto any food (you might want to start with oatmeal and salads).

Deep-Sea, Cold-Water Fish

- Anchovies
- Chilean sea bass*
- Cod
- Haddock
- Halibut*
- Herring

- Mackerel
- Salmon
- Sardines
- Scrod
- Swordfish*
- Tuna*

*not more than once a week because of mercury content

Nuts and seeds (including sesame, sunflower, safflower and all nuts) are generally the best sources of omega-6 fatty acids. GLA and LA (linolenic acid) are also found in animal proteins (from grain-fed animals), full fat dairy products (from grain-fed animals), shellfish, primrose oil, borage oil and black currant oil. Walnuts contain both omega-3s and omega-6s, the only nut to do so. Peanuts are really legumes rather than nuts, and as such they don't have much to offer when it comes to EFAs. I recommend avoiding them altogether, anyway, because peanuts are one of the most common foods people are allergic or sensitive to. Besides, unless you have organic peanuts, they come with the risk of contamination by aflatoxin—a waste product of mold, which is highly carcinogenic.

We get a lot of exposure to omega-6s—poor-quality omega-6s—from the meat we eat from grain-fed animals, which we must counter by getting plenty of both high-quality omega-6s and omega-3s.

Oh, Nuts!

To get the most nutrition, choose only raw, unprocessed nuts and seeds. Processing results in altering the good nutrients. You can get the benefits of the healthy fats from cold-pressed nut and seed oils, though you don't get the full nutritional impact of the whole food.

Keep oils (which should be cold pressed) tightly covered and store in a cool, dark place to prevent oxidation. Overheating oils or exposing them to light and air can change them into useless or harmful substances (like trans-fatty acids), make the oils rancid, and result in the exact opposite type of product you are trying to increase in your diet.

Grains have both omega-3s and omega-6s; it depends on the grain. (Grains also have protein as well as fat.) Corn contains omega-6s but is too starchy to eat a lot of. Corn oil is not a good choice either, mainly because the vast majority of what is sold does not provide good quality omega-6s, isn't organic, and shouldn't be used to cook at high temperatures. Sunflower oil is to be used for higher temperature cooking. I don't recommend canola or safflower oil either. The other oils (olive, walnut, pistachio, etc.) are used for flavor after cooking, or for very-low-temperature and short-term cooking. Cooking destroys the good properties of most oils.

Pat

Over the last year or two, Pat's weight, blood pressure, sugar levels and cholesterol kept rising (Syndrome X) while her thyroid levels fell—all of which
concerned her, of course. But what finally made her take action was the pain
she was getting in her knees—it got bad enough, often enough, to be lousing
up her golf game. Her doctor offered a panoply of medications and, after
some lobbying, a referral to a by-the-numbers food pyramid nutritionist. Pat's
numbers (her weight, cholesterol and golf score) kept climbing.

So I jotted down for her the basic tenets of the way of eating described in
this chapter. Once she started eating the right foods, the weight simply
dropped off. With no calorie counting, Pat lost twenty pounds in less than
two months! She didn't increase the amount of exercise she got, either—just
stuck with walking the golf course about twice a week and through her
neighborhood some evenings. Best of all, she told me (having been around
the diet block before), she was eating so much food! She was never hungry!
Her blood pressure and cholesterol improved as well. And her knees didn't
bother her anymore. On the downside, she's got no more excuses for those
high golf scores . . .

Drink Up

Perhaps the simplest step of all to nourishing your knees is to drink lots of water. The body consists mostly of water. It is vital for washing away the debris from all the chemical reactions that take place in the body and helping eliminate environmental toxins and pollutants, any of which can cause inflammation if left in the body. Also, cartilage needs plenty of water to keep it moist. It provides the lubrication necessary for the cartilage to allow a smoothly gliding joint. So drink lots of it, sixty-four ounces or more a day, preferably between meals.

Your other best beverage bet is green tea. Whether you drink it hot or iced, you'll get lots of anti-inflammatories as well as antioxidants. I recommend sipping it all day long. It is naturally low in caffeine, so you won't overload your body with stimulants. (And, if you switch to green tea instead of coffee, you'll avoid a host of other harmful components therein as well. In any event, you should keep your coffee to no more than one cup a day.)

You are better off without fruit juice—which concentrates the sugar and dispenses with the fiber—but if you can't do without it altogether, try mixing it with seltzer for a fruit juice spritzer.

Finally, vegetable juice is a great way to "drink your veggies," as long as you use the entire vegetable (so as to still get the fiber). Choose something other than canned juices, as they are generally full of salt. If you can find something fresh and organic and unsalted, that would be a reasonable choice, though best will always be what is made right in front of you, so you control the quality of what you eat (or, in this case, drink).

Foods to Avoid

In general you want to steer clear of refined and processed foods. Beyond that, avoid sugar (including honey, maple syrup, fruit juices and fruit concentrates) and simple carbohydrates, which provoke a rapid and prolonged insulin response that can cause stress, especially when it is chronic, and results in an increase in the production of inflammatory cytokines. Sugar in any form (which simple carbohydrates such as white flour and white rice are directly and immediately processed into) is also directly linked to weight gain, in part because what you don't use for energy now gets stored by the body, which hangs onto it as fat. Simple carbs also lack the micro- and macronutrients of their unprocessed predecessors, complex carbohydrates. Look out for even 100 percent whole wheat pasta—it is processed into simple carbohydrates during manufacturing. I want to note that you should avoid all rice, even brown rice for the first few weeks or months. (You can add some brown rice back in once you move beyond craving carbs.)

Avoid partially hydrogenated vegetable oils, which are present in many if not most commercially prepared baked goods, among other things, as they lack the nutrients and phytochemicals of healthy fats and have harmful trans-fatty acid properties to them.

Avoid the foods you are allergic or sensitive to, as they provoke an immune response that can cause skin changes, headaches, digestive troubles—and joint pain and swelling. The most common culprits are cow's milk and dairy products, sugar, wheat and peanuts, although responses are very individual and there is no need to avoid these foods if they do not bother you. The reactions to these foods can be delayed up to four days, so you don't always know what you are sensitive to. If you have suspicions (because maybe you have many types of unexplained symptoms that don't add up to a disease), you can be tested for IgG antibodies to see if certain foods are a problem for you. Although all doctors learn about these antibodies, by and large they don't think of them in connection to food sensitivities, so you may need to see someone who practices holistic, complementary medicine. Be warned—most insurance companies won't cover the testing, and your doctor will need to send the tests to special labs to get it done.

Finally, watch what you drink. More than a tenth of Americans' calories today are from the sugars and corn syrups in sodas, juices, teas and "sports drinks." Liquid sugar is the fastest of all into the bloodstream, so drinks such as these hold the biggest potential to wreak havoc on your blood sugar, insulin levels, and weight.

You should also avoid excessive alcohol. It interferes with blood sugar regulation as well as with calcium and magnesium metabolism, which is vital for strong bones. It is also high in mold, a common allergen. Keep it to under five regular-sized drinks a week.

Supplements

I believe that if you are perfectly healthy you probably can get all your nutrients from perfectly selected food. But who among us is perfect? So I recommend some basic supplements—food in a capsule—to my knee-pain patients, mostly to fight inflammation and ensure availability of the nutrients they need. These include: vitamin B_5, vitamin B_{12}, vitamin B_6, vitamin C with bioflavonoids, calcium, magnesium, zinc, copper, manganese, glucosamine, chondroitin, and omega-3 and omega-6 fatty acids. Key nutritional supplements and combination products will be covered in Chapter Nine.

Digesting It All

Good digestion and absorption are crucial in order for your body to take advantage of the good things you are feeding it. Furthermore, your digestive system and your immune system are intimately related. For example, bacteria in the bowel that help break down food can also create or destroy toxins, vitamins and other chemical substances. Whether they help or hurt you and your immune system depends on the health of your digestive system (as well as your liver, which detoxifies the body). Autoimmune illnesses and symptoms (including arthritic knees) can be greatly influenced by diet and by the health of your digestive tract.

Up to about 60 percent of the body's total immune system is found within the bowel walls. When foreign substances (such as infectious agents, toxins, pesticides, antibiotics, heavy metals, foreign hormones, pollutants and foods we are sensitive or allergic to) enter the body, the body perceives them as a foreign invading threat and produces antibodies to attack the foreign antigens. Sometimes when the immune system destroys a bacteria or virus, a toxin is released, triggering an immune response of its own. Or, if for some reason the body does not acknowledge that the battle has been won, it mounts a stepped-up attack, creating ever greater amounts of immune complexes (antibody-antigen combinations) that eventually, instead of remaining inside the bowel, start to get absorbed back into the bloodstream. There, they can move to various parts of the body, including, of course, the joints in general and the cartilage in particular. You know this as rheumatoid arthritis, lupus, psoriasis or just knee pain. (Avoiding the foreign substances that kick off this deadly cycle is one big reason organic food is best.)

The crucial relationship between the immune system and the bowel is another reason why NSAIDS are problematic: Long-term use can interfere with the health of the digestive system.

Having good digestion is also important for hormone balance. Estrogen metabolism is greatly influenced by bowel function and liver detoxification—these are important for absorbing and processing nutrients needed to form and balance hormones.

To ensure good digestion—as well as healthy bowels and immune systems—start by eating right. (And continue by dealing with any parasites and using probiotics and enzymes as described below.) It may sound simplistic, but chew whatever you eat well. Chewing sends signals that gear up the entire digestive system. There was a study of patients with feeding tubes placed directly into their stomachs, through which they were fed liquefied, nutrient-balanced meals. They quickly became malnourished. When they were asked to chew gum (so they would go through the motions of chewing) and given the same meals through the tube, those same patients were able to process the food and did not become malnourished.

Digestion *should* begin in the mouth, but it can't when you gulp down your food. Each step of the digestive process is carried out in specific organs, and only those organs. What is only digested in the mouth won't also get digested further along its path. If something doesn't get digested and properly processed upstream, it is useless everywhere downstream.

The human digestive and immune systems haven't yet fully evolved in everyone to successfully deal with sugar and refined grains, which is why those foods trigger allergy or sensitivity in so many people; if you are one of them, do yourself a favor and avoid these foods. Modern agriculture is very new in the scheme of human development. Sugar and refined grains didn't exist when Mother Nature began her work on us. Genetically and enzymatically, we as a species are evolving much more slowly than the food supply is changing. Not all of our bodies have quite gotten the hang of processing certain foods yet.

Parasites

Be sure you do not have abnormal bacteria or parasites living in your bowel wall. Ten percent or more of apparently healthy people are found to have parasites in their colon wall, though most doctors won't think to look for them if you don't have dysentery. Standard lab testing finds only a small portion of cases anyway. When I am suspicious a parasite may be present but conventional tests don't turn up anything, I suggest traditional testing done at labs that specialize in parasites. It's effective, but certainly not pleasant: you take something that gives you diarrhea; you then have to collect up the entire contents of your specimens for analysis—and you should do this three times (on different days)! This method, thorough though it seems, will still miss some cases of parasites. If the tests are negative or if a patient doesn't want to go through this, I have alternative methods that I do in my office or send to labs that do testing in different ways. Many practitioners of holistic medicine have methods of testing beyond regular labs.

On the plus side, if parasites are discovered, prescription antibiotics or herbs, or both, combined with nutritional support, almost always clears it up—along with whatever symptoms (like, say, painful knees) you were experiencing because of this hidden root cause. I always look for parasites in patients with autoimmune symptoms and/or illnesses. And I usually find them. It's not uncommon to be able to trace current problems back to an episode of food poisoning or a twenty-four-hour bug, often many years back, when the undetected parasites took hold. It is extremely rewarding to the patient and to me when symptoms and illness apparently unrelated to a process that began long ago are so easily eliminated.

Probiotics and Enzymes

Beyond the basic measures above, probiotics (healthy bacteria normally present in the digestive system) are always useful to good digestion and good health, and will be very important if you have immune problems affecting your joints. The bacteria break down all kinds of substances, which helps the body get access to nutrients as well as begin processing toxic substances. (Having a healthy liver, too, is important for detoxifying efficiently.) Poorly broken down substances leave debris that is toxic to our joints and to our bodies.

These probiotics grow on their own in a healthy digestive tract. But many factors can deplete your supply, including poor nutrition, diarrhea, antibiotic use or antibiotics in food, too little fiber in your diet (these bacteria use fiber as their nutrients), pesticides, toxins, viruses, parasites and exposure to bacteria from outside our bodies. You can restock with yogurt (check the label for "live cultures") or, for heavier lifting, supplements. If you do use supplements, make sure you get a balance of the types of bacteria that live in the small and large bowel—lactobacillus, bifidosporins, acidophilus and others—with labels promising you somewhere in the billions of organisms.

You also need prebiotics, which is the fiber the probiotics munch on and use to aid their work on your digestion. To ensure that they get what they need, make sure you get enough fiber, and a balance of soluble and insoluble fiber. (Soluble fiber, from oat bran, barley, nuts, seeds, beans, lentils, peas, some fruits—including apples, strawberries, and citrus—and many vegetables, slows digestion and helps the body absorb nutrients from food. Insoluble fiber, from whole grains and vegetables, helps food pass through the digestive system and adds bulk to the stool.) You can also take fructo-oligo saccharides and gamma orozonals, both prebiotics available at your health food store. You can also buy prebiotics and probiotics in combination capsules.

Finally, you need to have the proper enzymes throughout your digestive tract—and there are various types in the mouth, stomach, pancreas, small intestine and large intestine. Organ disease or dysfunction from any cause, including chronic illness, immune battles and infection, will deplete one or more of these enzymes. If you don't have enough of the enzymes that are supposed to be in the mouth, the digestion that is supposed to begin there doesn't, and the undigested food goes down into the stomach unprepared. The stomach enzymes, which can't do the mouth's work, will then only partially digest the food it is presented, and some debris will be left behind and passed through as the digestive process continues. That's assuming you have the right enzymes in the stomach. If you don't, the (ever larger) buck gets passed to the small intestine, where more debris is created, and so on. Furthermore, if you don't have the enzymes to properly digest the food, you won't be getting the nutrients you need out of your food no matter how good your diet. You'll also experience reflux, gas, bloating, cramps, and less than optimal bowel movements. Ideal would be to have a normal bowel movement after each meal. The pressure in the gastrointestinal tract is supposed to be equal from mouth to rectum. When you eat it should stimulate the process of moving the nutrient supply train—what goes in should result in an equal amount coming out. We are taught at a young age to "hold it in," and some have learned to have one morning bowel movement a day. While this is most usual, it is not, I believe, most normal.

If you suspect enzyme deficiency, supplements can help. I recommend a mix of digestive enzymes that does *not* include stomach acid (HCl) to begin with, taken at the end of your meal. The larger the meal, the larger the dose of enzymes you need to digest it, perhaps one capsule for a small meal and three for a large one. I think these are very safe, and I often recommend them. In cases of reflux, add deglycerinated licorice, taken before meals. If those steps don't cause a big improvement within a week or two, you should add the HCl and see if this helps you. I use betaine HCl, which is taken with meals.

Cynthia

Knee and foot pain would have seemed to be the least of Cynthia's problems, though they were severe enough to make it difficult for her to walk and impossible for her to exercise. Whatever was going on in her body even affected her brain function: She was depressed and paranoid, to the point where she'd been institutionalized. In addition, she had a ferocious case of psoriasis—an autoimmune disorder—so when she ended up in my office, the first thing I added to her long medical record was parasite testing. It came up a strong positive.

After all these many years, and many and varied doctor visits, the solution was simple: a short course of prescription antibiotics, combined with a long course of supplements and herbs, including horseradish, cloves, oregano oil and leaves, wormwood and other anti-parasitic herbs, probiotics, and EFAs, for normalizing bowel function and making the gut inhospitable for parasites. With the parasites gone, her immune system could be nutritionally repaired, and she recovered over a few months' time. She's certainly never needed inpatient services again, and she's mentally sharp, physically active, and griping about occasional small skin rashes that she once couldn't even have noticed amidst all the other chaos in her body.

It turns out that about eight years before she walked (well, hobbled) through my door, Cynthia had spent a couple days stuck in her bathroom with a vicious case of food poisoning. The symptoms started slowly as malfunction, not diseases, and progressed in intensity and frequency and severity. More and more functions became impaired until a diagnosis of rheumatoid arthritis and psoriasis was finally made. That's a fairly typical history for a patient with an immune disease. Here's the kicker: One of Cynthia's closest friends is an infectious disease specialist; he never so much as mentioned the possibility of infectious parasites to her. Take that as just another lesson on the importance of health-care providers who can see you as a whole person.

No-More-Knee-Pain Menus

This should be a simple way to eat. Eat whole foods, many different colors of fruits and vegetables, get a lot of fiber and increase your unsaturated fats over saturated fats. Reduce or eliminate sugar and simple carbohydrates. Drink a lot of water. It may take some getting used to, depending on how different if is from your current diet, but the general guidelines above should be all you need. This isn't a precise or complex system; it doesn't need to be. But it may seem overwhelming right now, as you contemplate putting it into practice. So I'll help you get started by giving you a week's worth of sample menus. There is nothing magic about the exact foods included here, and you'll notice that for the most part I haven't specified quantities. If you don't like salmon or collard greens, have halibut and spinach. If you like to have the same breakfast each and every day, go for it (as long as you have a variety of foods the rest of the day). If you don't have Tuesday's ingredients in the house, pick something you do have on hand until you get to the grocery store. If you're going out to eat, you should be able to find something on just about any menu that fulfills these guidelines.

Use these menus so you don't have to think about what to eat, if that's easier for you. Or, if you are the kind of person for whom that sort of rigidity is hard or you enjoy creating with food, then use these menus as suggestions only, and take off from there. In short, approach this program in whatever way makes it most likely you'll enjoy it—and stick with it! This isn't a "diet" but a way of eating—for life.

(As you look over these menus, keep in mind that snacks, too, are very important. You should have, in addition to the meals below, frequent snacks throughout the day, suggestions for which follow the main menus.)

MONDAY

Breakfast: Organic "old-fashioned" oatmeal with cinnamon, nuts or ground flax seeds; the oil of your choice; chopped apple, banana, pear or berries; and soy milk

Snack

Lunch: Egg salad (with chopped veggies and chopped apple, with olive oil replacing mayo, and seasonings and fresh herbs of your choice) served on a bed of lettuce with tomato wedges and cucumber slices

Snack

Dinner: Tuna steak topped with mango salsa served with roasted yams and steamed broccoli

Snack

TUESDAY

Breakfast: Twelve-grain bread with almond butter and a handful of mixed berries (whole or chopped) or sliced fruit on top

Snack

Lunch: Large mixed-vegetable salad topped with any combination of fish, grated organic cheese, chopped hard-boiled egg, seasoned baked tofu, beans and sunflower or sesame seeds, dressed with olive oil–based dressing and served with rice cakes

Snack

Dinner: Grilled free-range steak with sliced tomatoes with basil, and greens sautéed in olive oil with garlic

Snack

WEDNESDAY

Breakfast: Fruit smoothie with a protein whey or soy powder added

Snack

Lunch: Salmon burger with lettuce, tomatoes, sprouts and pesto sauce on a bed of arugula with a bowl of vegetable soup

Snack

Dinner: Thai curried vegetables over brown rice

Snack

THURSDAY

Breakfast: Organic plain yogurt (cow or sheep or goat or soy) with berries and ground flax seeds or nuts, sweetened with stevia, perhaps with whey protein powder added

Snack

Lunch: Three-bean chili and sautéed zucchini with lemon and olive oil

Snack

Dinner: Roasted chicken with rosemary, roasted veggies (cauliflower, brussels sprouts, beets), and mixed chopped-vegetable salad

Snack

FRIDAY

Breakfast: Eggs any way you like (using EPA- or DHA-enriched eggs—sometimes called omega-3 eggs), with soy "sausage," one slice twelve-grain toast with flavored olive oil, and half a grapefruit

Snack

Lunch: Chopped salad with chicken, apple, cashews and cabbage, dressed with pistachio oil

Snack

Dinner: Artichoke pasta primavera and mixed-greens salad with cauliflower, cabbage, broccoli, carrots, string beans, onions, etc., dressed with olive oil and garlic

Snack

SATURDAY

Breakfast: Lox and (a small amount of) organic soy cream cheese on whole-grain black bread, rye crisps or a twelve-grain bagel with the dough scooped out

Snack

Lunch: Scrambled eggs with salsa in a sprouted wheat tortilla with black beans

Snack

Dinner: Chilean sea bass with grilled onions, a variety of grilled vegetables dressed with olive oil, and spinach salad with mandarin oranges and almonds

Snack

SUNDAY

Breakfast: Omelet with onions, peppers and mushrooms, and sweet-potato hash browns

Snack

Lunch: Mushroom barley soup and sliced avocado and endive salad with lemon

Snack

Dinner: Free-range turkey burger smothered in onions and mushrooms sautéed in olive oil, steamed green beans and baby carrots flavored with mustard, lemon or organic butter

Snack

Now for those snacks. If you have a carbohydrate, try to eat it with a little protein and/or fat—for example, fresh fruit and a handful of raw nuts or seeds. Other good choices: a small piece of organic hard cheese; some hummus or baba ganoush with raw veggies; unsweetened granola with nuts; a hard-boiled egg; a protein shake (with fresh ground flax seeds); roasted garlic, or almond or cashew butter on a rice cake or celery stalk; lean, organic meat with mustard.

When eating meat or chicken, choose a small portion (you should get only three to six ounces a day; a four-ounce serving would be about the size of a deck of cards). With fish, a larger piece is fine. Eat your fill of any and all non-starchy vegetables, opting for fresh when possible (though frozen is acceptable). Add a large, green leafy salad to just about any of these meals—or all of them! Experiment to figure out the various greens you like, throw on as many veggies as you want (or have on hand), add some protein (beans, chicken, fish or tofu), and toss it with a dressing of your favorite oil (a good time to get in some more flax) flavored with lemon juice, vinegar, mustard, garlic, spices, soy sauce or whatever suits you. The idea is "nutrients in a bowl."

Nourish Your Knees

With smart food choices, you can eat your way right *out* of knee pain. This plan isn't designed with weight loss in mind—it doesn't specify portions or calorie counts, for example—but odds are this way of eating will get you to (or help you maintain) a healthy weight. This plan is good for all your body systems, not just your joints. To top it all off, it fights the inflammation at the heart of most knee pain. Nourish your knees this way, and they'll serve you well for a lifetime.

6

Move It or Lose It

Exercise in general is good for your whole body, but what's more newsworthy is that it's also good for preventing and reducing knee pain in particular. In almost all cases, the last thing you should do for knee pain is what most of us *do* do: Give it a rest. Staying in motion is one of the most important things you can do to keep your knees healthy. To get and stay pain-free, you need general conditioning to build cardiovascular endurance as well as balance strength, coordination, and flexibility throughout your body, combined with exercise aimed directly at your knees. Exercise (specifically appropriate strength training) is much more effective against knee pain than medication alone could ever be; it can help even when drugs have failed to. The more appropriate work your leg muscles do, the less of a burden your knee joints carry, and the less wear and tear there will be. Furthermore, muscles burn the most fuel, and the larger the muscle mass—and the larger *your* muscle mass—the more fuel burned, and the more weight you will lose, even when *not* exercising. Move it or lose it, I always say, with the second "it" being the easy use of your knees.

You should also move it *to* lose it, with the second "it" being excess weight. Exercise is important to general health and fitness, of course, and being healthy and fit can only be good for your knees. Being over-weight puts undue strain on your knees. Because of the type of joint the knee is, the force you place on your knee with weight-bearing movement can be three to four times your body weight. Among many other good things, maintaining a healthy weight protects your knees against a major stressor.

General health is the first level on which exercise is important to ridding yourself of knee pain or, better still, preventing it in the first place. The next level of exercising away knee pain is to add exercises specifically designed to protect your knee, to keep it functioning well and pain-free. You can think of it as "move it to lose it, part II," with the second "it" being knee pain. For the most part, this is going to mean some form of strength and coordination training, and Chapter Ten includes a sample program that fits the bill.

Specific exercises tailored to your particular situation can improve and maintain strength; increase or reestablish coordination between brain, nerves and muscles; and repair damaged tissue to restore normal function. The idea is to reverse the abnormal condition and reestablish a correct normal. You have to unlearn any and all bad habits before you learn new ones. In fact, you *shouldn't* strengthen until you learn those new patterns, otherwise you'll just strengthen bad habits and make any imbalances worse. The right program can help get your knees working good as new again.

The third level of exercising for the health of your knees is to learn techniques specific to whatever exercise you do, not only to improve your performance overall but also to do it safely in general, avoiding knee problems in particular. You'll also need strategies specific to what your mechanics and problems are.

Exercise can cause or exacerbate knee pain if done incorrectly or inappropriately. If you already have significant knee pain, it is a good idea to work with a physical therapist or knowledgeable certified fitness trainer at first. That will make sure not only that the exercise is safe but also that it is designed for your body in particular, with your specific limitations and goals in mind.

There is one time you should rest your knee because of knee pain, and that's if you have an acute traumatic injury. Even then, rest only for a few days to be sure it is stable. Do not "rest" your knee until it is entirely healed—it won't work anyway. Rest it until you are sure that the danger of creating further damage has passed, and then start using your knee.

Yes, I'm telling you that even though your knee hurts when all you're doing is standing up from a chair or walking down the hall, you should be hitting the gym. Even people whose knees have gotten so bad that their range of motion is limited should get their exercise. You need exercise to help your knee even if your doctor doesn't mention it. If patients think to ask, most are just told to walk, which is fine as far as it goes—it just doesn't go very far. The more you move, the better you feel, even when exercise is difficult at first because of knee pain.

A painful and sore knee will get stiff and weak if you just rest it. Resting will also alter nerve impulses and brain connections. In trying to protect the painful area, the brain turns certain muscles off and tightens others. Anticipating pain each time you move changes the normal brain-to-muscle communication. Some muscles underperform, others overcompensate, and, all in all, normal movement patterns are undermined. Over time, it will no longer be just your knee that hurts, but also other parts of your body. The way you step may change, the way your spine moves, the way you hold your head: Your whole body will be affected. Instead of resting, or limping, it is far better to protect what's hurting you by walking more slowly, conscious of how you are moving, with a normal gait, maintaining normal patterns of movement as best you can. You'll benefit most when your brain focuses conscious and unconscious thought on wellness rather than on anticipating pain.

So exercise, or keep exercising, unless you are in real danger of doing more damage. The trick then is knowing what's at risk. Very generally, if you experience real, exquisite pain when you bear weight on or move your knee, or you can't bend it at all without severe pain, or your knee locks and you can't straighten it—something gets stuck—you know something is urgently wrong. If you see a lot of black and blue, you can be sure something has been torn or seriously damaged. If every time you try to use your knee it swells and gets more painful, or if the joint is hot, you should have it checked out. These are all warning signs that you should not exercise until you've been examined and advised by a health-care professional. (Bear in mind that none of this necessarily means you should not exercise now, or never exercise—but you do need to think it through with someone experienced in such things.)

If, on the other hand, you fall into the far larger group of women with knee pain that is more of an ache, perhaps enough to make you limp, exercise is most likely to *help*. As a rule of thumb, if you can exercise, and as you do your knee loosens up and feels better, go ahead and exercise. Start slowly and work up toward increasing levels of exertion. If, however, you get worse as you move, get examined before continuing. Listen to your body; don't give in to your fears.

Moving your knee lessens pain and stiffness. Sometimes there's a direct effect, as with arthritis, the pain of which generally decreases as you increase your activity. Too much exercise or inappropriate exercise is not helpful. Rest just stiffens you up again. That's why your knees may be painful when you first get up in the morning or after you've been sitting down for too long—the joint simply hasn't been moving. When your knee is still for an extended period, the sinovial fluid on the joint surfaces between two bones gets compressed and absorbed into the cartilage. The bones move closer together, and when you do start to move the knee, there's not enough fluid to lubricate the joint. As you move, you'll get the fluid to all corners of the joint, and the lubrication eases the stiffness. But if you continue not to move, the joint, including the cartilage, dries out. (Poor nutrition and inflammation also dry out the joint.) When you are exercising, in any given session you'll generally loosen up as you go on, and your knee will hurt less. Furthermore, aerobic exercise has been proven to reduce pain in general by improving circulation of oxygen and nutrients and increasing production of endorphins, nature's feel-good substances.

Over time the effects are cumulative: Appropriate exercise builds up muscle, increases flexibility, and improves alignment, relieving the pressure on the joint and vanquishing knee pain.

You need to break the cycle of inactivity and pain. For one thing, when you don't exercise because your knee hurts, you're likely to gain weight, putting more stress on your joints and creating more pain. For another, when your knee hurts, your muscles weaken quite rapidly (up to 40 to 60 percent of strength can be lost within days of a painful injury), and the weakness creates more stress on the knee, creating more pain. When confronted with pain, your brain turns off (inhibits) the muscle at the joint, inhibiting it from firing, which leads to muscle weakness. As far as your brain is concerned, if something hurts, it's not going to move it. In some cases, you may need professional help to disinhibit those inhibited muscles, but once you do, building your strength back up is key not only to getting rid of the pain that caused the spasm and weakness in the first place, but also to making sure that whole chain reaction doesn't hobble you again.

Although regular exercise is a keystone of maintaining healthy knees and preventing knee pain, some knee pain and knee injury, however, is the result of overuse, often from athletic endeavors. So it is important to do the right kind of exercise, in the right amounts, with proper training techniques to guard against injury.

Diane

Diane didn't believe in taking supplements, in acupuncture, or in anything alternative, and her nagging knee pain didn't change that. She'd made it into her fifties just fine without that stuff, and didn't intend to start now.

She'd fallen a while back, twisting as she went down and landing on her knees and hip, and one knee was soon swollen and painful. The official diagnosis she received when it didn't go away after a few days was chondromalacia patella and patellofemoral syndrome with a medial meniscus tear and strained ligaments in her knee.

Diane took Celebrex for a few months and got some relief from it, though she never really got well. Her knee still hurt enough that she had to walk gingerly, and was extremely cautious about any physical activity. Then one weekend when she felt up to it, she went for a hike—and came home with a significant flare up of pain and stiffness in her knee.

That was enough to send her into physical therapy, where she had phonophoresis and ultrasound treatments, and did stretching, proprioceptive exercises and neuromuscular reeducation with her therapist. On her own, she also followed the therapist's instructions for walking on the treadmill and doing a modest strengthening-training program using some weight machines, some free weights, and some resistance bands.

Within six weeks, even on this less-than-extensive regimen, Diane was back to 100 percent. Actually, she told me, she felt better than she did before the injury. Though she'd done almost nothing in the way of exercise before her knee saga began—she belonged to a gym but never went, in case that sounds familiar to any of you—this experience inspired her to continue working out, gradually progressing, for the health of her whole body.

Science Says . . .

Studies abound showing that exercise improves joint health. As long as it is done with good form, staying active helps you create and maintain strength, flexibility and overall health. There are some holdouts, even in the medical world, who fear that exercise, or at least intense exercise, can further damage a sore knee, but there is little scientific evidence supporting that theory. The work being done on the issue shows just the opposite, in fact, and I'll touch on just a bit of it here to give you the general idea.

Studies aplenty show that people with osteoarthritis who follow an exercise program designed to eliminate knee pain get better pain relief and greater improvements in general functioning than patients who don't exercise, whether they work out alone or in a class, at home or at a gym, or in physical therapy, as long as the exercise program focuses on symmetric strength (appropriate strength in all the muscles that support the knee), balance, and muscle coordination, in combination with an aerobic component (generally walking).

Some research shows that for rehab after a knee injury, classes may be more effective than a home workout. But other research documents pretty much equal results in those who work out with a physical therapist and those who are on their own, at home, working with very basic equipment and little supervision beyond initial instruction to ensure good technique and sufficient challenge. Of note, though not particularly surprising, is that the more closely participants followed the prescribed exercise regimen, no matter where they did it, the better their results were. Exercise doesn't work if you don't do it!

No doubt different people react to different situations differently. My advice is to ask yourself if you would benefit from the supervision and peer pressure and/or support of a class. Would it make you toe the line for a more intense workout? Would you be motivated to actually do the workout, if you had a class or appointment blocked out on your calendar—or had already shelled out the money for it? Or would you be more likely to exercise if you could squeeze it in at any time of the day or night, without worry about gym hours or going out in bad weather? Does just the thought of the gym intimidate you, so you would be more likely to exert yourself in the privacy of your own home? Do you compare yourself negatively against others in a class or would you take inspiration from others' efforts? You know yourself best; pick whatever strategy—or combination of strategies—will make it most likely that you not only begin an exercise program but also stay with it.

A study done in England demonstrated that when patients with osteoarthritis got relief from their knee pain (in this setup, via injection, into the joint, of a local anesthetic or a placebo—with similar results!), the strength in their thigh muscles increased. What's most interesting to me about this is not so much what it tells us about the possible benefits of injections but how important the link between pain and strength is. Instead of no pain, no gain, no pain *brings* gain. I heartily recommend strength training to relieve pain in the knee; I'm intrigued by the promise of the cycle that may start—that of lessening pain allowing for more gains in strength, which in turn reduces pain further, and so on. (I also find fascinating what is revealed about the power of the mind to heal, as demonstrated by a placebo performing equally well as a drug, but that's another story.)

Taking off from studies showing about 70 percent of patients with decreased knee pain and improved knee function within 6 to 8 weeks of beginning an exercise program, another researcher boosted the results further still by adding exercises designed to improve balance and coordination to the more usual strength training. More than 80 percent of those patients were good as new with this training, and able to resume all their regular activities, including sports, with no pain, or almost no pain, at their original level, if not better.

A study done at Tufts University medical school, which was published in 2001 in the *Journal of Rheumatology*, found that patients with knee osteoarthritis who did strength training decreased their pain, on average, 43 percent, and improved their physical function 44 percent, while a comparison group managed only 12 percent and 22 percent respectively. The program involved exercising at home with inexpensive equipment, with initial instruction but no ongoing supervision.

Biomechanical Stress

So despite the people, including doctors, who think exercise, or too much exercise, is actually a risk factor for osteoarthritis and knee pain, in reality healthy knees will withstand even intense, long-term—low-impact—exercise without pain and without incurring OA at any greater rate than non-exercisers, or any earlier, or any worse. (High-impact exercise, such as running, can increase knee strain and damage proportional to the degree of weakness and mechanical errors involved.) Some people with old injuries and certain biomechanical issues need to take special care about the type of exercise they do, and they need to be careful about how they do it, to avoid an increased risk of OA and injuries. But then, so should everybody.

Overuse of the knee (your muscles and knee should never feel more than a little fatigued after a workout) can increase the risk of OA and knee pain, and biomechanical stresses can also cause joint damage. Prime among those stresses are muscle weakness, or unevenness in the strength of related muscles, and poor muscle coordination. Their effects may go unnoticed in younger people, but the truth will come out in older bodies. The good news is that these stresses are entirely preventable with proper exercise. You might not be able to change all the anatomical issues that can cause biomechanical stress on your knees, but we know how to address and compensate for many if not most.

The most common biomechanical stress of all on your knees comes from being overweight. And, in fact, women with osteoarthritis in their knees weigh, on average, about 15 percent more than those who are free of the disease.

It makes intuitive sense that someone carrying around too much weight on their bodies might have sore knees. What may be less obvious is that someone of normal weight but with weak muscles will put the same amount of stress on their knees as an overweight person. When excess weight and insufficient muscle strength meet, then you really have a problem. People who weigh more generally have more muscle mass, which you might think would be good. But those muscles, sizeable though they are, don't generate or absorb as much force as the somewhat smaller muscles in people who are not overweight. Large muscles don't always mean strong or healthy muscles.

The way female bodies are put together versus the way men are built can also mean trouble at the knee. The main difference here is that women's hips are wider in relation to their knees, resulting in their knees being relatively knock-kneed, which puts more mechanical stress on the knee.

Neuromuscular Control and Proprioception

The key to prevention of (and recovery from) knee injury and pain are neuromuscular control and proprioception (feeling where the parts of your joint are in relation to the rest of your body), both of which are crucial for joint stability. Increasing your neuromuscular awareness will bring improvements in balance, coordination and strength—and reduction in risk of injury or likelihood of pain. Proper training protects your knee from inappropriate force and excessive stress.

The neuromuscular differences between men and women surely account for at least a portion of women's greater susceptibility to knee pain and many knee injuries. Unless specifically trained to do otherwise, women tend to move in ways that stress the knees. Women rely more entirely on their quads in situations of physical exertion such as playing sports, jumping, and even standing and balancing, whereas men also put their hamstrings into play (stabilizing the knee); women land jumps with their legs stiffer and straighter, and with more rotation in the hip (when landing on one leg), meaning the soft tissue of the knee absorbs the impact of their full body weight (instead of the muscles engaging and stabilizing the joint), putting more stress on the knee. (This helps explain why most knee injuries in women, even women athletes, are "noncontact," and involve landing a jump or pivoting while jumping to change direction.)

On top of that, women tend to have somewhat less leg strength, less endurance, and slower muscle reaction times than men. For instance, women's hamstrings are usually slower to work up to their maximum power when they are exercised. Women more often have strength imbalances, poorly synchronized muscle timing—which muscles initiate movement and which ones follow to complete the movement—and uneven muscle usage and coordination. Most people have unequal strength in the various thigh muscles; women in particular have strength in the front of the thigh that overshadows the side and back muscles. That type of asymmetrical muscle development can interfere with knee mechanics. When you bend your knee, the kneecap might get pulled one way or the other rather than tracking correctly up and down, and put abnormal pressure on the various shock-absorbing and stabilizing tissues of the knee joint.

Many women with osteoarthritis also have weak thigh muscles (quadriceps)—15 to 18 percent less strength than women without OA. That's generally been thought to be a result of a painful knee getting little use, so that the muscles atrophy. But I agree with the experts' re-thinking of the equation to consider that muscle weakness might be the *cause* of knee pain, rather than the result—that is, the chicken, rather than the egg. If your quads are weak, there's going to be more uneven pressures on the knee any time you stand or walk, which could, in the end, lead to wear-and-tear arthritis (osteoarthritis).

All this means that women's knees are just generally less stable than men's are. Their motor control strategies create more opportunity for injury. Just think of what you mean when you think of someone as running "like a girl" and you'll see how different patterns of movement can be. Unlike some anatomical differences we just have to live with, muscle imbalances and the like are easily corrected with exercise. Neuromuscular training—working not just on the strength of your muscles but also on how your muscles work together—will help you keep your knees stable, no matter what activities you decide to engage in, and also reduce your risk of injury.

Plyometrics is one key type of neuromuscular training. The most common form is jump training, which is designed to make you stronger and help you jump higher. But what's so crucial about it is that it helps you learn to control your leg muscles and stabilize your joints throughout a jump, so you can minimize the force of impact on your knees when you land. Athletes in sports that call for a lot of jumping can stave off injuries as well as improve performance this way. But what would be good for Mia Hamm, or your teenage daughter who idolizes her, might also be good for you, even if you never do more at a soccer match than pace the sidelines.

One study compared female volleyball players before and after they did a jump-training program against men (who didn't do the training). After training, the women's landing force from a block jump decreased 22 percent, and they had half the number of instances of torquing the knee—performing better than the men on both counts. The women who did the special training ended up correcting imbalances in muscles strength on the dominant and nondominant sides of their bodies. And, their average jump height increased 10 percent!

Researchers training female athletes in injury-prevention techniques for as little as four weeks were able to dramatically reduce the number of knee injuries (essentially bringing it down to the same rate as men's). Women who didn't get the neuromuscular and jump training had more than three times the rate of injury of women who did.

A similar study of nearly 3000 female soccer players showed that specialized neuromuscular and proprioceptive training reduced ACL injuries by 88 percent. This program focused on how to "run, jump and pivot like boys," as one of the investigators put it—that is, with knees bent, and lower to the ground than girls, who tend to keep their legs stiff and stand upright when they play. Training involved a thorough twenty minute warm-up period of stretching and strengthening (especially the quads and hamstrings), jumping drills, instruction on avoiding injury (how to land from a jump, for example), as well as exercises specific to the sport, using no extra equipment and with an emphasis on proper technique, done two to three times a week for three months.

How to Exercise

There is no one specific exercise, or type of exercise, to get rid of or stave off knee pain. Aside from avoiding high-impact exercise such as jogging and high-impact aerobics, what specific exercise you do matters less than that you just do it—and do it properly. Mix it up (cross train) to keep yourself interested and challenged, and to avoid over-stressing your knee in any one particular way. Make sure your chosen activities are intense enough for your muscles to feel a little fatigued, and that they encourage strength, flexibility, balance and alignment along with cardiovascular fitness. Some things hit many of these points all at once (such as yoga, tai chi or qi gong), but variety will work for you with your own individualized cross-training program. Whatever you do, do it right (i.e., safely—see below). And pick things you like, so that you'll actually *do* them—and keep doing them.

Good technique is always important in preventing injury, and especially so if your passion is soccer, basketball, tennis, or some other sport that is notoriously tough on knees. Learn and practice safe ways to jump and turn. (See "Exercising Safely" at the end of this chapter.) And you should always warm up your muscles before exercising at full capacity with a few minutes of walking or riding a stationary bike, or going through the motions of whatever you are about to do in a slow and easy fashion until your muscles are warmed and ready to serve and protect.

As purely a matter of health and well being—and reaching and maintaining an ideal body weight via an efficient metabolism—you should also do at least half an hour of aerobic cardiovascular exercise four times a week. Your target heart rate should be 70–80 percent of your maximum predicted heart rate, which you can estimate by subtracting your age from 180. You should not be breathing so hard that you can't carry on a conversation with someone next to you. You can divide up the time you spend exercising, walking fifteen minutes to and from work, for example.

What is known in the trade as "skill training" or "functional training" covers three types of skills important to your neuromuscular system: strength (which accounts for not only how much force your muscles can produce but also how much they can absorb); balance (maintaining a stable center of gravity); and coordination (between nerves and muscles, timing muscle contractions, as well as between groups of muscles). Lest you be tempted to gloss over that last one, let me point out that all conscious movement—and most things you need to do to get through your day—involves rather complex coordination, which most of us take for granted. You need efficient give-and-take among your body's muscles, and among muscles and nerves, to function smoothly. Just standing on one foot (say, to begin climbing the stairs) requires your nervous system to orchestrate opposing muscles to lift one leg, support the other, and stabilize the torso all at once. No matter how strong you are, without that synergy you can't even do that one simple action. The idea is to coordinate your nervous system with your muscles and even your bones so you can move efficiently, smoothly and with purpose—and without pain.

For both strength and coordination, it is a good idea to train groups of muscles all at once, rather than each muscle in isolation, at least some of the time—that is, to use your muscles when you exercise the way you use them in life. Except perhaps when you are using a weight machine, real life never requires you to work just your abductor, or just your adductor, or what have you—your brain fires off instructions to groups of muscles when it wants something done well and efficiently. By the same token, you want to focus your training—even when you're aiming at your knee—not on the one joint but on the whole leg and, in fact, on the whole body. They're all in it together.

Chapter Ten gives you guidance on specific exercises to do to help you plan your own exercise routine.

Throw in some proprioceptive training, and you'll really be on your way. "Proprioceptive" is the technical term for a sense of spatial relations within the body, and of the body in space. Just where is your foot in relation to your knee? In relation to the hill you're climbing? Any kind of exercise focused on balance will improve your proprioception. The best examples are sitting or laying on those large rubber Physioballs, and working out on balance or wobble boards. I like the way these activities combine strengthening, coordination and balance.

When designing an exercise plan for yourself and your knees, you have to take any other medical problems you have into account. But even patients with serious conditions of most types improve with exercise, though they may require a more structured program or closer supervision. If you're dealing with any significant health concerns, you should check with your doctor before taking up exercise (if you are a recovering couch potato) or beginning a new form of intense exercise (even if you've been exercising regularly).

Even people with serious or long-term knee pain should notice clear results from exercise in short order. Everyday activities such as climbing stairs, getting out of a car after a long drive, and putting on your socks will be easy again. Like Ella (in Chapter Two), it may be that the physical problems in your knee don't vanish with exercise, but that the pain does.

Even if you need surgery, exercise is critical to getting the best results. Getting in shape before (and after) surgery, especially if you're having total replacement, will ease and speed your recovery and up the odds of your knee fully functioning in the end. If a limp has become your normal pattern of walking, you'll tend to keep doing that after surgery unless you intervene with proper training. After surgery, putting weight on your knee actually aids in recovery, which is why rehab usually includes walking and strengthening exercises along with stretching.

Qi Gong

If I had to choose one physical activity that would be best for your knee, I'd have to say traditional Chinese qi gong. Although I'm introducing it primarily as a form of exercise, qi gong is really an entire preventative health-care system unto itself, and has been so used in Eastern medicine for more than thirty-five hundred years. With its gentle movements, combined mind-body awareness for intrinsic stress-reduction as well as direct physical benefits, I can't recommend it highly enough.

Qi gong works on the assumption that mind and body are inextricably linked. It is a holistic exercise, aimed at making the wall between the conscious and subconscious mind more permeable, allowing energy to flow freely to all parts of your body. (This is the basis of all Eastern healing.) Before it starts to sound too "out there," let me emphasize that qi gong builds strength, flexibility, balance and coordination. It recognizes the importance of posture, stance and alignment, all of which are key to knee pain—not to mention overall well-being. It will help you lessen friction in your joints, preserving healthy cartilage and bone.

Relaxation is a key principle of qi gong, and it includes the specific idea of relaxing and opening the joints. Movement is difficult if joints are tense, and your muscles will be tense as well; in addition, you'll be open to the possibility of irritation and inflammation in the cartilage. Relaxation means more than just releasing tension, however. In a truly relaxed state, you will not only be supple but also alert and quietly active.

Qi gong considers the joints to be gateways for the qi, or energy, and emphasizes keeping the gateways open by learning to relax and release the joints consciously. Emotional and/or physical stress leads to tightened muscles and from there to restricted joints. "Relaxing open" the joints—relaxing and opening the joints to qi (that's the Asian phrase you'd hear)—helps qi to flow, which helps *you* to flow—not just in terms of moving fluidly but also in terms of seamlessly integrating all aspects of your being (body, mind and spirit) and bringing your own best self to the fore.

Many of qi gong's precepts are beginning to edge into medical practice, a tiny trend I certainly hope will continue. A few years back, I went to visit my brother Robert Kessler, who is also an osteopathic physician, in Boulder City, Nevada. He was all excited to tell me about a great continuing medical education course he had just taken. He said it was the best approach to exercise therapy he had ever seen, and totally different from the familiar sports-medicine approach of focusing work on one muscle or muscle group at a time. This new approach used many parts of the body at once, combining functional strengthening (making muscles stronger in ways in which you use them in real life, as opposed to just when you are at the gym) with proprioceptive training and neuromuscular reeducation. His instructor emphasized how the program could change the way muscles were working, and the way they were communicating with other muscles and with the brain.

My brother began to show me some of the exercises he'd learned, but I stopped him midway to show *him* something: a qi gong program I teach to my patients—the same one I do myself. The movements combine strength and balance and relaxation, it takes me only about ten minutes, and every joint and muscle in the body moves. My brother was amazed to see how similar it looked to what he had just learned, and told me that my regimen covered everything he saw in the course, though in a different sequence. Not that it was billed that way for this group of mainstream physicians, but the "new" approach my brother learned was clearly derived from thirty-five-hundred-year-old traditional Chinese medicine, such as qi gong.

Qi gong can be done by anyone at any level of physical ability and at any level of intensity that you wish. A qi gong workout can be done sitting in a chair or, as when my associate Dr. Ka does it, it can be a seriously intense martial-arts workout that is incredible to watch. I teach a sort of junior high school version most everyone can do—a beginner's program that should be useful your whole life. The basic program is just a series of six exercises—though each has probably about twenty moves in it. For specific health problems we will sometimes add one or two more sets of exercises.

Qi gong and its subtleties are best learned from an instructor, live and in person, rather than from a book, so I'm not going to give you "Qi Gong for Knees" here. Qi gong has increased in popularity in recent years such that in most areas of the country you should be able to find a class near you, at least to get you started. If not, or, if you prefer to do it on your own instead of or in addition to a class, plenty of good videos are available, and there are many books devoted entirely to the subject as well. A good course will teach you the sequence of the motions, and when those become automatic, so you can do them without thinking, you can continue on your own at home if you like. (Or, by all means, continue with a class if that's more inspiring to you.) Once you're in that qi gong zone, and you no longer have to consciously focus on the physical movements anymore, you'll also start benefiting from the meditative component of this kind of exercise.

I would like to give you a few very basic principles I've learned in my own practice of qi gong, which I've carried over into all kinds of physical activities. I think you'll find them helpful whether or not you ever learn a qi gong movement: Consciously try to release tension in your shoulders, fingers, hips, ankles and toes in particular. Keep your wrists soft, and don't lock your elbows or knees. Imagine your vertebrae are supple, like a rope. Try to think of your joints relaxing open, with a gentle expansion from their centers, and be aware of places you tend to contract inward. Think about oxygen, blood and energy all moving freely with no obstructions or tensions hampering their flow.

Exercising Safely

What you need to do to exercise safely depends on your level of conditioning and the exercise you are engaging in. But everyone needs to be aware of it. Consider this: Your knee takes the force of your entire body weight (at least) with every step you take—and three times your full weight when going up stairs. That's a lot of stress. A few simple strategies can make it as easy to bear as possible. For women in particular, here are some of the areas to be aware of, getting more specific as we go:

- Get regular exercise. Working out infrequently puts you at greater risk of injury—that means you, "weekend warrior," playing racquetball twice a month only, or jogging only when you're near a pretty trail.

- No matter what else your exercise routine consists of, include stretching, balance improvement, strength training, and jumping.

- Stretch before and after you work out, no matter what kind of exercise or sport you choose. You should stretch your whole body, with particular attention to your pelvis, hips, thighs, legs, feet and ankles to benefit your knee. Tight leg muscles are a setup for injury. If you don't like to stretch before exercise, then warm and prepare your muscles by doing the activity you will be engaging in for a few minutes much more slowly before going full out. But stretching afterward is a must.

- Build up your leg muscles in general, in order to spare your ligaments. Jogging and jumping (done correctly) are especially good for this.

- When you jump, take off and land on both feet. Landing a jump puts seven to ten times your body's weight on your knees, and the only way to ease the burden is to share it.

- Land jumps with your knees slightly bent, on the balls of your feet, with your weight on both feet evenly, rocking back to the middle of your foot. Don't land flat-footed or with your legs stiff.

- Strengthen your hamstrings specifically. Run backward; jump; "rebound" (mini-trampoline); do leg presses, squats, hamstring curls, lunges. Women tend to overrely on their quads (in the front of the thigh) without integrating the gluteals and hamstrings (in the back) the way men do, and miss out on that additional stability.

- Improve your balance. Stand on one foot. Jump rope. Hop. Play hopscotch! Walk a balance beam (real or imagined). Do tai chi, yoga, or qi gong. Dance. Try a balance board or a Physioball.

- Try working out in the water, where your natural buoyancy takes pressure off your knees. It's a sure bet for preventing knee pain, and it is especially useful for exercising when your knees already hurt.

- Crouch slightly. This should be your neutral position in many sports, but women tend to adopt a more upright position.

- When you bend your knees, make sure they point straight ahead, moving right out over your shoelaces and not in toward each other or out to the side. Keep them working like the hinges they are (and not like ball-and-socket joints). Be especially careful when you pivot or change direction. Don't let your knee twist. Don't begin a turn with your knees—start with your head and your knees will follow.

- Stop with three little steps instead of one sudden stop ("plant").

- Make sure you wear appropriate, supportive shoes.

Get Moving

With these general concepts in mind, you are ready for the specific workout plans in Chapter Ten. Whatever way you stay active, have a good frame of mind and be positive. Being healthy is a wonderful gift you can give yourself. Enjoy it and have fun.

7

I Can't Stress This Enough

Physical, psychological and emotional stress can all cause joint pain. Although we view stress as an emotional thing, we have a very physical and physiological response to stress—we hunch over, clench our muscles, raise our blood pressure, speed our heart rate, and slow our digestion, among other things. That much you are probably aware of by this point. A tension headache is the most famous sign of this kind of tightening of your muscles, but it can cause strain anywhere in the body, including the knees.

We feel stress when something threatens our survival instinct. Stress triggers the mobilization of stored energy reserves. Your blood sugar increases, fat breakdown and digestion slow, food and fat are called out of storage to be ready for use. Your adrenaline surges—the "fight or flight" response. In other words you are primed and ready to run from that saber-toothed tiger (once literal, now more often figurative) you face. When you don't use these processes productively—if you don't physically run away from the perceived threat, then rest and return to normal, or if you don't fight until certain victory—you're left with altered body functions, such as sugars that will be stored as fat, and fat that will be stored rather than used; inflammatory metabolic debris with an affinity for synovial joint fluids; and a condition that mimics insulin resistance. It is like packing for a long trip and then suddenly having nowhere to go. You're left with all these suitcases that you can either unpack right now in an orderly fashion or throw into the closet to do later, as you are already pooped from packing them. Most of us, unfortunately, tend to go for the closet.

Chronic stress, emotional or physical, also causes inflammation. And some of the hormones released to handle stress in turn release or create pro-inflammatory molecules.

Stress also influences gene expression. We probably all have the genetic potential to develop joint problems, including arthritis and knee pain. Some of us have more potential than others, it's true. But in any case, not everyone realizes that potential. The chronic release of those pro-inflammatory molecules can be what makes the difference. One way we can prevent the joint problems made possible by our genes is by limiting our exposure to those inflammatory molecules by limiting our stress or supporting our body's ability to respond to stress. We can also reverse a problem that has already appeared, by similar means.

Furthermore, stress creates anxiety and fear (again through hormones), which can make you eat more, or less, or less well, and so get insufficient or poor nutrients; it also slows the digestive process, therefore interfering with the absorption of nutrients. Additionally, stress increases the action of the autonomic nervous system's "speed up" section. (It has a "slow down" section too, for the record.) This leads to poor body fat distribution and poor digestion, and impairs the liver's ability to detoxify the body. Poor nutrition and/or high body toxins will eventually come home to roost in your joints.

Thoroughly tested psychological scales assign points to life events, both positive and negative, according to how much stress they bring—death in the family, new baby, getting fired, starting a new job, getting divorced, getting married, and so on. Studies show that people with the most points at a given time had the greatest negative effect on their immune system. They were the most likely to catch a cold or contract some other infection. True, you don't "catch" knee pain, but my point is that stress is physically very hard on your body, and it can as easily show up in your knees as in a runny nose or headache.

Caroline

Caroline is a high-powered executive working seventy hours a week. She exercised seven days a week, running hard and pumping iron when possible. She ate reasonably well, although she often missed a meal and frequently ate on the run. And she hurt all the time. Her muscles were tight. Her joints ached.

Her constant stress was to blame. Her long hours were one obvious physical stress, and she was actually over-exercising, too, which created more stress on the body. She lived with quite a lot of emotional stress as well, always feeling she needed to prove to herself and anyone else who was watching that she was a rising star and, to boot, that she was never going to grow old. For her, it was all about being "number one." When you are number one, there's nowhere to go but down, and living with that ever-present anxiety is extremely stressful. Caroline's stress was also upsetting her hormone balance, which was not helping her joint pains.

Fortunately for her, the solution was fairly straightforward: fine-tuning her diet to be more nutritious, and especially to include anti-inflammatory essential fatty acids, berries and cruciferous vegetables, all of which she chewed while seated and relaxed; cutting back on exercise, keeping it to four days a week of a somewhat less rigorous program; and, finally, taking time in the middle of each marathon workday to close the office door, turn off the lights, mute the phone—and meditate. For half an hour, each day, Caroline visualized herself and her place in the world in a positive way, the way she'd like it to be. It was a really long thirty minutes at first, but gradually she learned to lose herself in that small oasis. She told me she found it brought her new perspective, and reliably took the sting out of the crisis of the day. Within a few months, her joint pain had completely reversed itself, and she had much more time to live her life instead of just going along for the ride. Her work improved, her life improved, and she didn't hurt all the time.

Stress and Hormones and Knees

Whether any given stress is physical or emotional, the process remains the same. When you are under stress, your body releases adrenal hormones, including adrenaline, cortisol and DHEA to handle it. Chronic stress can exhaust the adrenal gland's ability to respond appropriately, and eventually deplete your body of certain crucial hormones. This creates hormonal imbalances that can negatively affect the knee (among other things).

Without enough DHEA and cortisol, not only can't your body mount a response to stress but it also can't mount an anti-inflammatory response. Insufficient DHEA exaggerates the imbalance of estrogen, progesterone and testosterone, which, as we've seen, can lead to inflammation in the joints. Low levels of cortisol, the body's main anti-inflammatory hormone, can result in increased aches and pains, including knee pain. High levels of cortisol are also unhealthy for the bones and connective tissue.

Low levels of cortisol may be another reason you may wake up with stiff and sore knees. Anti-inflammatory cortisol levels normally peak in the morning, but with chronic stress, you don't have enough cortisol to keep that up, and you're then on your own to face the effects that little motion through the night has on your joints. This effect is exacerbated if you are not getting restful, restorative sleep, or not getting enough of it. The lack of sleep in itself is a stressor, and drains your stress hormones. Besides, your body normally uses the "down time" while you are asleep to repair itself as needed, including the joints, and lack of quality sleep means you go without this necessary basic maintenance.

Stress can also change the way hormones are converted in the body. Your body converts the stress hormones into sex hormones (estrogen, progesterone, testosterone). This is the normal process, but it works both ways—sex hormones can be converted into stress hormones. If the body converts sex hormones into stress hormones to handle an overload of stress, you'd suffer from insufficiency or imbalance of those sex hormones, which, as discussed in Chapter Four, can cause joint problems.

By the way, all of these hormones are made from the basic hormone called cholesterol. I heard a story at a conference about a woman who went to a research center to have her hormones measured via a blood test. As she was backing out of her parking space afterward, she had a fender-bender with another car. She wasn't hurt, but she was shaken up, and she went back inside and asked if she could have a glass of water and sit for a moment. The doctor asked if she would allow him to redo the blood test to see what effect the stress had. Just fifteen minutes after the first test, with nothing additional to eat, her cholesterol was *100 points higher.* When her body needed more stress hormones, it produced more of the raw material (cholesterol) it needed to manufacture them.

Finally, hormone levels influence how women perceive pain, how they handle it, and how they respond to treatment. Hormone levels affect your mood, and your mood affects your response to pain. Low estrogen levels, for instance (which can be brought about by stress), are closely linked to depression, since estrogen promotes the synthesis of mood-stabilizing neurotransmitters such as serotonin. When stress ruins your hormonal balance, you are more likely to feel pain (any kind of pain, including knee pain), feel it more intensely, feel less able to cope with it, and respond less completely to any intervention.

On the flip side of all this, stress reduction can be a huge help in relieving pain, as the next chapter will explore further. Getting rid of stress, or learning to manage it productively, will also help balance your hormones, thereby reducing inflammation and eliminating knee pain, along with relieving many other unwanted symptoms. See Chapter Four for a more thorough look at hormones and knee pain.

Camilla

Camilla was perfect. At least she worked very hard to be. Perfect mom, perfect wife, perfect friend, perfect neighbor. Not to mention running her own business—perfectly. She worked very long, very intense days, always intent on producing the highest quality work. She ate perfectly, too—or so she thought—carefully monitoring her fat intake to keep it very low and to keep herself thin. She tried to be physically perfect too, running nearly every day and doing yoga several hours a week as well, all of which she thought was necessary to be in perfect shape.

Camilla's knees, however, were not perfect. They hurt her, and she had pain in her other joints as well, along with osteoporosis, although she was only fifty. She also had high cholesterol, despite her "perfect" low-fat food pyramid diet. She finally wound up in my office because none of the ten or so other doctors she'd been to over the years could figure out why she was losing bone mass at her age, with her attention to what she ate and her level of fitness.

I did a lengthy workup, and discovered that, in scientific terms, Camilla was stressed out! Her cortisol levels (the body's primary response to stress) were sky-high. I didn't really need the blood work to tell me that, however. Plainly, her quest to be perfect took quite a toll on her. She pushed and pushed, sacrificing herself to everyone and everything that was important to her. She was always on the go, always doing something. She had no quiet time, no room on her agenda for personal time, no tolerance for the occasional selfish action. With all she was giving, she had nothing left over to heal herself.

Even the measures Camilla took to take care of herself—diet and exercise—were fraught with pressure. Not only was there the mental and emotional stress of feeling she had to do them *right*, all the time, but those healthful impulses themselves were actually bringing physical stress to her body. She was stoking insulin resistance with her low-fat, high-carb diet, and she still craved sugar and starches constantly. She ran harder and longer and farther when she recognized she was stressed out, pounding her knees and setting the bar ever higher for herself in the process. Even her "relaxation" was stressful: an intense form of yoga in a class full of competitive types.

My prescription was for a new way of eating, a new way of exercising, and a new way of relaxing, all aimed at helping Camilla de-stress her life. I recommended an eating plan such as the one in this book, designed to deal with her insulin resistance, helped along by supplements as well as other nutrients aimed at cholesterol metabolism. I actually suggested she cut back on her exercise, running limited amounts at limited speed, and not every day. I told her a walk or slow jog would, for her, be even better. I recommended an Iyengar yoga class, in which poses are held for several minutes each, with the goal of relaxing her body into each position, letting the energy flow through her body, breathing well and fully. And, perhaps most important of all for Camilla, I encouraged her to make room for a special quiet time for herself a couple times a day. The assignment was a tough one for her, even harder than cutting back on her running: Sit still. Be quiet. Do nothing. For a few minutes at a time, create quiet within yourself, find a way to get centered.

With this plan in place, Camilla returned to the care of her regular physician and I didn't follow her case directly anymore. I'm happy to report, however, that several months later her doctor was impressed enough with her progress to call me to let me know how well she was doing.

Autoimmune Diseases

Besides wreaking havoc with your hormones and thus on your knees, stress affects the immune system in another way. When your body is confronted by a foreign substance, such as an infection, heavy metal or any kind of pollutant, it thinks it is under attack and produces antibodies in response to the detected antigens. In a common immune system misperception, the body often confuses an invading antigen's protein with the similar protein in the body. If the similarity is to cartilage, then the body attacks its own cartilage. Together the antibodies and antigens form an immune complex, which often makes itself at home in the cartilage. This is what happens in autoimmune diseases, a category that includes rheumatoid arthritis, lupus, and psoriasis (which can affect the skin or the joints, or both). Even if the antibody-antigen battle commences on your skin (as in eczema or rosacea), in your nose (as in rhinitis), or in your stomach (as in colitis or Crohn's disease), the effects of it may well be felt in your joints, including your knees.

Before it gets bad enough to give it a name and call it a disease, the process of this kind of reaction in your body may still produce symptoms. That stiffness in your knee when you wake up could be the first signs of that battle. The way I explain all this to my patients is to ask them to imagine their husband has a cold. That cold virus is an antigen, and his body produces cold antibodies; they do battle, the antibodies win, and the cold goes away. Now, perhaps he was kind enough to share that cold virus antigen with you. But instead of cold antibodies, your body crosses its wires and produces cartilage antibodies. In vast quantities. Even when the cold virus is gone, your body still perceives a threat to your cartilage from the antigen. And especially if you've got a genetic predisposition to arthritis, it won't be long before all this shows up in your knees.

This "cold" could be the trigger that makes you realize the potential of your genetic predisposition. Just having a gene for something does not mean we're going to *express* the gene. A study of identical twins showed that at least 70 percent of what accounts for incidence of breast cancer was environmental. That is, people with identical genes did not get breast cancer at identical rates; the difference was in how they lived and what they had been exposed to. This is wonderful news: Even if you have a gene for arthritis or some other knee problem, you have control over whether or not it ever shows up. If you keep the right kind of environment around you and your knee—nutritious foods, lots of water, clean air, plenty of oxygen from exercise, and so on—you control the fate of the gene. Even once a gene has been expressed, there's evidence we can reverse that expression, repair the gene or alter the effect the gene has. The bottom line: You may be right to be concerned about your knees because of your mother's or sister's or grandmother's experiences with her knees, but you are definitely not condemned to repeat them, even if the two of you share the genetic code.

Mind-body techniques are very helpful with autoimmune illnesses because of their intimate connection to stress, and I recommend them to you as I do to my patients. Keep in mind, however, that they may not be sufficient to solve the problem on their own, and you'll need to get to the root cause to rid yourself of it entirely. Whenever a patient of mine has many symptoms but they add up to no one disease, I always look for an autoimmune response—and whatever is triggering it.

Mood and Knee Pain

Knee pain can be depressing, but this is a bit of a chicken-and-egg situation. Having your knees hurt every time you take a step may well get you down. Arthritis, for instance, is linked with increases in depression and anxiety. But this works the other way, too: Depression can create or exacerbate knee pain. Muscles react to the way we feel. Depression often involves changes in muscle tone throughout your whole body—the familiar slumped shoulders, head-down posture, with the muscles in the face sagging. Depressed people physically *look* sad, and contracted within themselves. That posture will impact your knees sooner more often than later. Anxiety, too, can play havoc with your knees. And improving your mood can be enough to cure your knee pain. It is not mind *over* matter but simply that the mind *does* matter. Think of how you felt—how your body felt—some time when something wonderful happened to you. I'm betting you got over that nagging cold, or your headache stopped pounding—or your knees no longer hurt.

My Wrist Bone's Connected to Your Knee Bone . . .

Everything I need to know about stress and knee pain I learned from my wrist. Not the factual, scientific stuff, of course, which I got from journals and research, but the everyday, real-life experience of the link between stress and pain that let me truly understand (and so, successfully address) what so many of my patients were going through. Of course, as I was living through it myself, it took awhile to realize what was going on in my own body, despite my almost daily discussions of parallel problems with my patients.

I hurt my wrist while golfing with a friend of mine who is a far superior golfer. I was down in a sand trap, and swung hard to try to get 180 yards onto the green. My club hit the edge of the sand trap after it connected with its intended target, and the pain was immediate. I couldn't even finish the hole, let alone the course.

I saw a series of doctors and received a series of vague diagnoses. None of them found anything specifically wrong with my wrist, though I was in enough pain—on my dominant side—that it was interfering with basic daily activities. I tried physical therapy, with phonophoresis (current and heat directed to specific areas) ten times and myriad exercise machines. I saw an acupuncturist a few times. I followed all the advice I give to my patients—eating well, taking supplements, exercising. But I wasn't getting better with all the things I recommend for everybody else. My wrist still hurt. This went on for three months.

On the links that day, I was taking a break from the several major projects I was in the midst of. All of them would be great for my work life—if they went well. But I was taking risks, putting myself out there, and facing, at best, some professional embarrassment if they didn't work out as I hoped they would. I recognized that I was under a lot of stress, but it didn't seem to me like more than I could handle. Whose work doesn't stress them out from time to time? It never occurred to me that there could be a connection to what was going on in my wrist.

Since nothing else was helping, I finally made an appointment with an energy healer in my office. Why not? I was ready to try anything to get easy use of my right hand and arm back. She held my hurting hand and wrist as we talked about what was going on in my life and my world. She made some observations about what we discussed and even some personal suggestions for me to think about, moving my hand to different positions as we spoke. As she explains it, she was clearing my energy fields, balancing the energy flow to and from my hand and all throughout my body. She also gave me some tools to keep the flow going myself.

The weekend after my session, after just one treatment, I was back on the golf course for the first time in months, playing with minimal pain. After a second session, I was pain-free.

It was only then that I was forced to consider that the pain in my wrist was a manifestation of my emotional state. Not that the injury wasn't real—it was—but I was holding on to the pain for emotional reasons. I knew I really hurt myself, but what if, as the healer suggested, I'd maintained the pain in my hand so that if everything didn't come out right, I'd have something to blame my failure on? With this realization—and the "unblocking" of my energy—my body could let go of the pain. I had to face my own little referendum on "how good a doctor do my peers really think I am?" on my own. And for good measure, "how good a physician and healer do I think I am?" These are serious issues which were being raised in my unconscious mind—and old and even childhood issues were being brought up and challenging me. It was much better to address the real issue than to focus on the pain in my wrist. (Though I have to admit, getting at the real stuff was probably harder.) Once I was resolved to do that, come what may, my wrist stopped hurting. Good thing, too, because I really needed the stress relief I generally find on the golf course!

Lessons from Finland and Beyond

You don't have to rely on touchy/feely stories such as mine or even Camilla's to find the link between stress and knee pain. I'll give you just one example from recent research that connects those dots quite clearly—and scientifically. Previous research has tied lack of job security—i.e., stress—with health problems in general. In the study I'm talking about now, Finnish researchers looked at a variety of chronic pain problems, including osteoarthritis and especially back pain, among government employees who remained on the job after many of their colleagues had been downsized. Those workers were under increased stress, both physical and psychological, from both extra work (covering for those who were no longer there) and uncertainty about their own futures.

Sure enough, employees working after major layoffs were five and a half times more likely to miss work because of pain problems than they were before the downsizing, and researchers found an increase in the rate of osteoarthritis, among other issues. People who had back problems to start out with fared the worst, but many with no previous problems developed pain too. And women were more dramatically affected than men. U.S. researchers in parallel fields suggested that the effects of job-related stress on pain is even greater in this country because job security is much higher in Finland than it is here, so the people in this study had little to fear, really, in the way of their own jobs once they survived the cuts. You could do a whole other study on those who were laid off and unemployed, and I bet you'd find increases in pain in that group too, from the stresses in their lives, but that's another story.

Though the Finnish team didn't ask participants specifically about knee pain, I think they could have, and come up with similar results. The main theme here—that major life stresses are closely linked with musculoskeletal problems—is what is important to our discussion of knees and how they relate to the whole body, and indeed the whole self.

8

Your Knee Bone's Connected to Your . . .

Just as postural imbalances can create knee pain, so can spiritual and emotional imbalances. Having a healthy knee requires a healthy body, mind and spirit. Pain in any of those areas can show up in your knee. That's not to say that "it's all in your mind." Your pain may be caused by bone or cartilage or muscles, or it may be caused by (or worsened by) emotions or stress, but still it is your pain, and you can be free of it. You deserve to be free of it.

Women are right to be wary of being told "it's all in your mind." The medical profession unfortunately has a bad track record when it comes to dismissing women's pain. And knee pain is a good candidate for this kind of dismissal, as many, many cases don't have the obvious hallmarks of any particular injury or condition. Too often, if a doctor doesn't know which box to check off on the insurance company chart, he'll just let it go at that. No specific diagnosis results in no specific treatment. But for the patient, the pain remains.

For women and men, knee pain can be caused or worsened by stress (as we've seen in Chapter Seven) or any other kind of mental, emotional or spiritual pain. Physical symptoms may well be linked to the psychological processes. Furthermore, it is well documented that faith, spirituality, religious belief and even prayer all correlate positively with health and healing. Calling on these parts of yourself can help you get and stay healthier.

Susan

I had one patient named Susan who woke up one day with excruciating knee pain that just wouldn't go away. Now, all the women in her family seemed to have knee pain, so she wasn't exactly shocked—except for the fact that her own knees hadn't bothered her before. But she had recently turned forty, and was feeling old and ugly.

She started with supplements and improving her diet, and within several weeks reported her pain was about 50 percent better—but still very much there. Discouraged, she abandoned her efforts, and her pain soon resurged.

Then came September 11, 2001, and Susan started to feel really out of control of her life. One of her responses was to refocus on her health and her body, and she cleaned up her diet again and resumed taking supplements. This time, however, she also began prayerful meditating. She described her practice as communing with a higher power she believed she could rely on, and placing faith in goodness and wellness, fixating on light rather than darkness. She wasn't a practicing participant in any organized religion, but she found it to be important nonetheless to identify herself as a spiritual person—and then take actions that let her put that into practice.

This turned out to be a really powerful combination. In less time than it had taken her to give up on eating right the first time around, her knee pain vanished. What physical changes alone couldn't accomplish, spiritual connection could.

Anything that reduces stress is going to improve the condition of your knees. There is plenty of science to show that meditation and prayer (even others praying for you without you knowing about it!) and other spiritual endeavors work on that level, along with guided relaxation, deep breathing and similar techniques.

A strong social support system has also been shown to ease and speed recovery from an injury and help with learning to handle pain, as has simply talking with someone in a similar situation to your own. Receiving empathy, feeling understood, and having a support system all help you maintain a positive attitude and channel negative feelings in as productive a way as possible—both of which have been well established as beneficial to your health and well-being. Studies show how this works by actually altering brain chemistry, as an antidepressant would.

One place the benefits of social support have been studied is in the context of AA (Alcoholics Anonymous), where it has been dubbed the "herding response." Research shows that people often go into a meeting feeling down and depressed, but after spending time in an environment in which everyone is supportive and empathetic, and in which everyone assures them, they can do it, they feel they can get through whatever they are facing. Those same people walk out no longer depressed. Talking and emotional exchange has changed the hormones in their brains, which in turn has changed their mood.

Women and men tend to have different ways of coping with pain. Despite the stereotype that women ("the weaker sex") are more susceptible to pain, studies show women are actually better able to handle pain. For example, a study done on arthritis patients showed that when rating their pain "high," women were more likely than men to use a range of ways of managing it. Their strategies included distracting themselves, relaxing, and turning to other people for emotional support. Following such a bad day, men reported being in a bad mood, but women didn't. Researchers concluded that by taking steps to be in control of the pain, women were able to limit its psychological costs more than men.

Our experiences and expectations of pain, even from earliest childhood, have a lot to do with how we handle pain in our lives today. We learn what pain means in many ways from early childhood on, and no doubt men and women are socialized differently in this regard. Dr. Ka, the doctor of Traditional Chinese Medicine who shares my office space, makes the connection to how women deal with pain from the contemplation of, preparation for, and experience of both the beauty and difficulty of childbirth. Most women are taught, often starting very early in their lives, that childbirth is the most painful thing. The implicit message that comes along with this is that to be fully grown up, fully a woman, they are going to have to learn to face and control pain. It's a woman's job, they learn, to deal with pain and still carry on (whatever the source of the pain).

Meta Messages

This chapter is about the power of the mind, and how to harness this power to use it in healing ways. If any parts of it don't appeal to you— particularly this section—you have my official permission to simply go ahead with what you learn in other sections and other chapters. But those of you who are tuned into this sort of stuff may benefit by considering the metaphorical messages of painful knees. (Thanks to Thorwald Dethlefsen's *The Healing Power of Illness* for insights into metaphysical aspects of illness, several of which are reflected among the aspects mentioned here.)

You are the only person who can rightly read the symbolic content of your symptoms. The ideas and associations here are meant *not* as some kind of decoder key—like those "dream interpretation" dictionaries that let you look up specific meanings of specific images—but rather as a source of associations to spur your own thinking on the subject. Not all of these (or even any of them) will be true for any given person, and the list is surely not exhaustive. While this pain has your attention, you may as well use it as a window into what is going on in your life, to be honest with yourself about *all* the things you are feeling.

None of this is to say you don't have a physical issue with your knee or physical approaches to eliminating the problem. But for many people, there is a subtext to their experience, and delving into it may prove fruitful. I've experienced it myself, with the wrist injury described in Chapter Seven, and seen it work wonders in countless patients.

With all that in mind:

Knees painful enough to interfere with our normal activities or mobility could be signaling that we need a rest; perhaps they are slowing us down because we don't seem to do so on our own. Unwanted outward stillness may be a call for needed inward stillness.

Knees are the primary source of your ability to move forward or up in the world. Problems in the knee can hinder your progress figuratively as much as literally; or, your knees may hurt because you aren't moving ahead, or are fearful of what lies ahead.

Strength requires flexibility, and here again this applies both literally and figuratively. If your knee is stiff and painful, perhaps you as well as your joint would benefit from gaining flexibility. Or, a certain stiffness in your personality may also be bothering you.

Because it is a joint—a crossroads, a coming together—the knee signifies connection. If you feel disconnected, that could well show up physically in a joint such as the knee.

Stiff knees could signify unhelpful rigidity somewhere in your approach to life: an inability to bend, or bend easily. Perhaps stubbornness sometimes gets in your way.

As it bends, the knee symbolizes the ability to choose between two directions or two states of being. So perhaps your aching knees are telling you that you need to stop and think about the choices you are making and the direction you are taking. Joint pain may be related to moments of change in your life.

Knee pain could be your body signaling you that you need to be able to kneel down before a higher power, to realize you are not the ultimate authority in the universe. Kneeling also represents humility, and anything making it difficult or impossible to kneel might be showing you a need to develop that part of yourself, curbing any tendency toward feelings of superiority. Or, looking at kneeling as a sign of dependency on others, knee pain could be encouraging us to allow ourselves to depend on others, loosening our fixation on a vision of ourselves as self-sufficient, and realizing we are just one small part of something much larger than ourselves.

On a related tangent, according to the principles of reflexology, knees represent pride and ego—and an injury there may well have come about as a result of an excess of those traits.

Aches and pains, including knee pain, are sometimes thought to be hurts you turned in on yourself to avoid hurting others. If you lash out at someone, they hurt—if you don't, you hurt. Women have a greater tendency toward this kind of bottled up aggression than do men—and a greater tendency to have hard-to-diagnose aches and pains—but both sexes can avoid physical manifestations of that pain by learning productive ways to channel their aggression.

Our knees quite literally support us in this world. Knee pain may mean you feel unsupported—or that you are not supporting yourself.

Similarly, through the lens of qi gong, knee pain, especially stiff or locked knees, may mean that you simply "can't stand" your current situation. With aching knees, you can't feel truly grounded. When we fear the very earth cannot support us, we are constantly attempting to somehow pull ourselves up and away from it, creating a physical strain on our knees and throwing us off balance. Locked knees, the argument goes, show an inability to trust.

Qi gong holds that this kind of pain, from stiff or locked knees, reinforces the wall between the conscious and subconscious mind, while the truest healing comes with fluidity between the two. Stiff, locked knees disturb our balance in a very fundamental way. Imagine trying to walk a tightrope with completely straight legs! But when the knees bend (as they do in all types of qi gong movement), we center ourselves. It's not just a physical centering but a spiritual one as well, helping us find a place where our core beings are in balance, allowing us to live at peace and with full awareness. Coming at it from another direction, you may find that focusing on what does help you feel connected, grounded, and aligned within yourself will rebound to the benefit of your knees as well.

Whether you are left or right dominant, and which knee your pain is in, may color your interpretation of what knee pain means to you. For example, if you are right dominant (right-handed), you generally step forward first with your right leg. Pain in the right knee may signal you to stop and evaluate before making a big change (moving forward in the world). If it is, rather, your left knee—your weight-bearing leg—that hurts, perhaps the signal is that your body is holding you back; it is not ready to support the change.

Even the language we use to refer to knee pain can give us insight into ourselves and our lives. The labels we give to our symptoms are often the key to understanding their symbolic meaning. Think about a knee that's "strained," "stiff" or "twisted." Or muscles that are "overworked." Or a joint that's "messed up" or "over-extended." We say we "just can't straighten out" a knee (or a situation, or a relationship . . .). Maybe a knee has "gone too far" or "been under too much pressure." Stepping back a little, we can also consider the dual meanings of words that describe our physical bodies as well as our attitudes. Starting with "attitude," as a matter of fact, and including "stance," "position," "posture" and more—all of which are seriously affected by knee pain. Here again, the outer mirrors the inner; the physical and psychic are linked like two sides of the same coin.

So ask yourself what your knee might be telling you. Ask yourself where you are going, what's in your way, what changes you may face, what choices are yours to make, and so on. Look inward, and answer honestly. Look at how you explain your situation to yourself and others, listening for clues in both your message and how you express it. It could be that changing the way you think about your knee pain will also change your knee pain or, at the very least, your experience of your knee pain.

If any of this resonates with you, you'll find it helpful to decode whatever message your symptoms have for you. You may also benefit by seeing a health-care practitioner who uses this type of an approach to health and healing. If it pains you to answer or address these questions honestly and fully, recognize that there is a problem that you don't have the tools to fix, and seek assistance from a professional—a therapist, a healer or any practitioner able to help you help yourself. When you find resistance in yourself but know somehow in the back of your mind that the issue is important for you, that's what you most need to pursue. It's by exploring those things that are not easy to recognize or easy to deal with that you will benefit most.

Johanna

Johanna's knee pain seemed to start out of the blue. It had never bothered her in the first fifty years of her life, and she hadn't been injured. But now her knee was killing her.

Closer questioning revealed that the throbbing in her knee began right around the time Johanna's company was thrown into chaos when a key employee quit and a major project ended. Her stress level was really ramped up.

In an attempt to quiet her knee, Johanna had tried a little of this, a little of that—homeopathy, Eastern medicine, and so on. But her pain finally resolved when she started working with a spiritual counselor to reevaluate her life. She realized that what was happening at work wasn't her. And it was still her business, and business was still good. Despite her feelings, everything wasn't, in point of fact, falling apart. The end of the project she'd worked on for years had left her feeling as if she didn't know where she was or where she was going—as if she had nothing to do and nowhere to go. So she figured out her new short- and long-term goals, and finally understood for herself that life simply goes on. By regaining focus on where she wanted to go and choosing her own direction, Johanna proved to herself that she wasn't helpless, and that she *was* stable.

"I went through this whole emotional thing of getting my feet literally back on the ground," she explains. Once she felt in control of her life again, that was the last of her knee pain.

The Power of Placebo

Some people will dismiss reports of knee pain relieved through psychological, emotional or spiritual work as all in the mind—along with the knee pain itself. But I happen to agree that you can think yourself right into knee pain—and that you can think yourself right out of it too. I think that's great. I say: Since the mind is that powerful when it comes to healing, let's learn how to tap into that power. We may not be making miracles, but I think the end result is something better: a real, complete cure that is within anyone's grasp.

The best medical science has long studied this phenomenon, though mostly while looking the other way. The research held in highest regard—the double-blind placebo controlled study—compares a group of patients receiving an active ingredient with a group receiving something thought to be inert (a placebo). The researchers are looking for the effect of the active substance, naturally, and more than three quarters of the time it does indeed outperform the placebo. But placebos turn out not to be truly inert; about 30 percent of the time, they equal or better the substance being tested.

Almost always, the effectiveness of the placebo is overshadowed by the success of whatever it is being compared against. But when you think about it, if roughly a third of the time the brain can make symptoms go away, isn't that great? Wouldn't it be wonderful if we could learn to harness that power? To induce it anytime we wanted? Reams of research show that you can, in fact, teach your mind to teach your body that it is healthy rather than unhealthy. With proper training, patients have been able to increase the success rates of mind over body to the point where they approximate the success rates of pharmaceuticals and other medical interventions. Harvard medical researcher Herbert Benson, M.D., famous for "the relaxation response," calls the phenomenon "remembered wellness."

Over the years, placebos have been show to affect just about any physical function you can measure. They've worked to some degree just about any time they've been tested. And they've worked not just transiently but for months or years. It's a powerful response.

Your Worst Fears

A recent study asked one group of people with chronic illnesses, including arthritis, to spend twenty minutes each day for three days in a row writing in a private journal about their worst fears. No one but the writer ever saw those journals. But people who spent that time recognizing what they were most afraid of, what fears motivated them, what fears affected their thinking and behavior, turned out to have far fewer problems from their conditions than people who didn't journal, or who did different kinds of journaling exercises. They had fewer symptoms and fewer outbreaks of symptoms, and needed less medication. Putting their deepest thoughts into words, bringing them from the unconscious to the conscious, dealing with them directly in this way, even for a short period of time, paid off over the long term.

We do have to keep in mind that it works the other way too, and some members of the placebo group always end up experiencing some of the side effects of the active ingredient being tested. Furthermore, studies show that, in short, thinking you are sick can be enough to make you sick. This is placebo's evil twin, "nocebo." The classic study of this effect dates back a hundred years, before we got so picky about the ethical issues surrounding *causing* illness in patients; it featured doctors inducing wheezing in allergic patients by showing them an artificial flower. A more recent study of this effect showed that women who believed they were prone to heart disease died at four times the rate of women who didn't think they were but had, in point of fact, equivalent risk factors. Still other research, this time of heart patients taking blood thinners (or placebos), documented the effect when one of the centers conducting the tests did not include in their protocol a warning to patients of possible GI side effects. Patients at the other two centers, who did receive the warning, were three times as likely to experience stomach pain.

We can learn something beneficial from nocebo, too, about our susceptibility to self-fulfilling prophecies, and the possibilities of worrying ourselves sick. You're not likely to get a lot of help for problems such as these from your garden-variety mainstream physicians, who aren't trained to handle what they've been taught to write off as psychosomatic. They've been taught to consider psychosomatic illness as a possibility in patients who have vague complaints that are hard to pin down with a single diagnosis, and those who are sure that whatever is prescribed won't help much, on the theory that low expectations are usually met.

From your position as a patient, the take-home message here is (a) to be open to the power of positive thinking, and (b) to work with a doctor you really trust to find a treatment plan you really believe in. When you and your doctor truly believe and expect that you will be well, chances are very strong that you will be well. Whatever the specifics of the approach you choose, if you have those things going for you, you are more likely to find success with it.

Herbert Benson, M.D., also studied the effects of what he called "belief and expectation," and found that most patients greatly benefited from nothing more than meeting three basic conditions: Patients have to believe and expect they are going to be well; doctors have to believe and expect the patient is going to be well; and patients and doctors have to believe in and expect the best from each other. Combined, those three things alone were enough to bring healing. Benson's studies showed effects of symptoms in an exhaustive list of conditions, including arthritis and pain.

That's how you make the power of placebo work for you (even if it is doing so in conjunction with physically active approaches). You can tap directly into placebo power using a variety of readily available techniques, including meditation, visualization and even chanting or sound or vibration therapy. There are many forms of each of these, and they can be easily explored (start with your local library, bookstore, health food store or wellness center). Again I'd like to say: It's not so much mind *over* matter, as it is simply that the mind *does* matter.

Sonya, who you read about in Chapter Three, provides a good example. An important step for her in getting rid of knee pain was to believe she could and would be well. She'd come to think of herself as having "bad knees." In that frame of mind, she moved gingerly, anticipating pain with each step, attempting to protect her knee and herself. But that only further entrenched poor body mechanics, which turned out to be the heart of her pain. Sonya needed to learn to move normally, if slowly, so she could get and keep her muscles functioning normally. Osteopathic manipulation helped her on this pathway, but another crucial factor was her attitude. Once she stopped approaching a staircase with only one thought in her mind—*"This is going to hurt!"*—she found she could, in fact, ascend without pain if she moved consciously, focusing not on potential pain but on a natural flow of movement.

Ella, from Chapter Two, faced a similar realization. After a few months on the program I recommended for her knee pain, Ella complained at her checkup that her knees were no better. And, in fact, I could see they were still large and swollen and ugly. When I inquired about the pain and stiffness in her knee, Ella reported it was greatly reduced, and indeed, she was now walking without a limp. She'd become so used to living with pain, and she so hated the way her knees looked, she hadn't even really noticed the pain receding! Ella had to appreciate the progress she had made before she felt healed.

Working Together

These may not exactly be topics your doctor brings up. The best health-care professionals of any type are "holistic," that is, they take the whole patient, and all aspects of their lives—body, mind and spirit—into account. This can be any traditional or alternative practitioner, whether a family physician, a surgeon, a dermatologist or any number of others. I think most physicians went into medicine with all the best intentions of healing people and diminishing suffering. In reality, however, the current medical system doesn't allow much time and space for that, with most traditional doctors working within the labyrinth of subspecialty-oriented medicine, insurance and managed-care regulations and paperwork. You may want to explore other avenues in conjunction with your regular health care, including reflexology, massage, acupuncture, bodywork, Traditional Chinese Medicine, energy healing, homeopathy, and osteopathic medicine (see Chapter Nine). But don't be afraid to bring these subjects up even with your internist or other doctor, and remember you always have the right to choose a different doctor if you don't like the response you get. You are in charge of your health, and you choose the supporting cast in the play that you are directing.

9

Natural Pain Management

Y ou'll find plenty of hype in any health food store about the latest and greatest substances for any imaginable ailment, and it isn't always easy to sort out fact from wishful thinking. But that's no reason to write them all off. With a little careful investigation, you can find many things there (or at a medical center or a spa) that you can use to rid yourself of knee pain.

In fact, you can probably find too many things. That's why the very best therapy would be a plan individualized to your particular circumstances. That's what you'll get from a good holistic practitioner, but it is more difficult to do with a book. Given that we're working with a single chapter of a book, I'm going to give you an overview of just some of the most generally effective approaches, then provide boxes summarizing what you should take, tailoring programs to three levels to get as close as possible to your specific situation. I don't want you to get overwhelmed by the size of the list of supplements I review here, though I do want you to be impressed by how much potential help there is outside of NSAIDs and other drastic measures. I am not suggesting that anyone take everything I cover in this chapter, or that you can only be well if you take all of them. Ultimately, you'll find most of these in combination products, so you won't be dealing with fistfuls of pills each day. By the end of the chapter you'll have specific guidelines on what sorts of ingredients, and in roughly what doses, to look for, and you'll be ready to shop for the best quality products in the most efficient combinations to cover the bases you need covered.

The body is constantly breaking down cartilage—and, ideally at the same time, constantly rebuilding it. So most of what's here are natural treatments that slow or stop the destruction of cartilage, or help with cartilage creation and repair, and diminish pain.

Vitamins and Micronutrients

If you follow the eating plan in this book, getting a wide variety of vegetables (especially cruciferous and green leafy), fruits (especially berries), nuts, vegetable oils, whole grains, beans and legumes, meats, eggs and cold-water fish in the process, you'll get all of the basic nutrients your body needs. For those of us with imperfect diets (and that's just about everybody I know, including me), supplements are a valuable insurance policy for overall good health. In addition, many vitamins, minerals and other micronutrients benefit your knees specifically, preventing and even relieving knee pain, including:

- **Vitamin A (beta-carotene)**, an antioxidant, improves immune function and thyroid function, and is needed to form bones and teeth.

- **B vitamins** act as coenzymes, among their many helpful functions and properties. They are needed for energy production and to maintain healthy tissues. B vitamins such as niacin (B_3), riboflavin (B_2), B_5 (pantothenic acid) and B_6 (pyridoxine) are important for forming collagen.

- **Vitamin C,** another antioxidant, helps promote healing and tissue repair in general. Specifically, it is a necessary ingredient for forming collagen, a protein (the most abundant protein in the body) needed to make the body's connective tissue, including the tissue in the joints. Take vitamin C with bioflavonoids to enhance its benefits, as they are also anti-inflammatory and antioxidant.

- **Vitamin D** also improves immune function and is needed for healthy bone and thyroid function. It is very important for growth and development in children.

- **Vitamin E** is another antioxidant, which prevents cell damage in the body and is helpful for tissue repair. The most common vitamin E sold in stores is D-alpha tocopherol, but I think that an E made up of mixed tocopherols and tocotrienols is the most beneficial and the only one to take.

- **Copper is** crucial for making and repairing cartilage.

- **Magnesium** helps make collagen and bone. It is essential for enzyme activity and in energy production.

- **Iron** helps make collagen. It is an essential ingredient for making enzymes and keeping the immune system healthy.

- Trace minerals, including **sulfur, chromium, boron, silica,** and **manganese,** are necessary for making collagen and bone. Manganese is important for making and repairing cartilage as well, and for protein and fat metabolism.

- **Zinc, selenium, beta-carotene, calcium,** and **chromium** round out the minerals and nutrients helpful for general joint health.

There are still other important nutrients. I could write a whole book, rather than a single chapter, on the subject. That's part of why a varied diet is so important—and why a good multivitamin/multimineral supplement is too. You should be able to find one that contains all or most of the above in adequate amounts. (See the box at the end of the chapter.)

Besides having individual effects on the body, vitamins and nutrients also help each other work better, so taking them together and in as complete a regimen as possible is important. For example, vitamin C and vitamin E taken together make each other more effective, and the body needs zinc to maintain proper levels of vitamin E in the blood.

Glucosamine and Chondroitin

Though all my patients use a multipronged approach to getting rid of knee pain, because no one tactic is going to work as well on its own as it will in intelligent combinations, if I had to pick one key supplement to combat knee pain, this would be it. These two substances are so often combined in a single product it is sometimes hard to sort out the effects of each, so we'll talk first about what we know about how they work together. That's the way they are most often used—the way I frequently recommend using them—anyway. But if you could only use one, it should be glucosamine, which I believe is the more important of the two.

Glucosamine and chondroitin provide pain relief and help heal and maintain cartilage. Both are anti-inflammatory, and are important components of the framework cartilage is built on. Used consistently, they decrease knee pain from arthritis and can even slow progression of the condition, according to a study published in the mainstream medical journal *The Lancet* in 2001. That's one of the best studies to date, if still on the small side. An analysis of fifteen solid studies published in the *Journal of the American Medical Association* in 2000 concluded that glucosamine and chondroitin effectively relieved symptoms of arthritis. It noted the flaws in the studies available to work from, but added that they weren't much different from the flaws in the studies done of NSAIDs.

Even the very conservative Arthritis Foundation and *Consumer Reports* have been convinced. We'll know still more when a large-scale (and very expensive!) study currently underway at NIH (National Institutes of Health) is completed in 2005, comparing glucosamine and chondroitin with both Celebrex and a placebo.

I recommend these supplements to just about every adult over thirty-five and everybody who has joint pain.

Be aware, however, that glucosamine and chondroitin are both large molecules unlikely to be absorbed through the skin. I believe that you have to ingest them to reap their benefits. That means the plethora of creams being hawked with these as key ingredients are probably charging extra for ingredients that at best won't work efficiently topically (though they may be combined with other ingredients such as topical analgesics that may help).

Glucosamine, which the body makes on its own, serves as a key building block in making cartilage, and in helping the cartilage retain moisture. Glucosamine also relieves inflammation and tenderness. Glucosamine supplements, unlike NSAIDs, go beyond just reducing symptoms, however, to actually slowing the progression of damage to the joint. Glucosamine appears to stimulate cartilage cells in the joints to make proteins joints need for smooth functioning, may help prevent collagen from breaking down, and protects joints from further damage by allowing water to remain in the sponge we call cartilage. This improved lubrication decreases the wear and tear on bone that eventually gets labeled osteoarthritis.

Studies have shown glucosamine to be more effective at reducing joint pain and improving mobility than a placebo, and, over time, at least as effective as anti-inflammatory drugs such as ibuprofen as well as standard anti-arthritis drugs. In studies done over three years, people who took glucosamine not only had the same or less pain and stiffness than those who took prescription medication, but also had much less cartilage loss, as shown on X rays, than those who only took prescription medications in the class of drugs called NSAIDs (which includes ibuprofen, aspirin, and cox-2 inhibitors such as Celebrex and Vioxx). In fact, the NSAIDs group kept losing cartilage, while those in the glucosamine group had no loss—or even an increase.

This is an enormously helpful supplement. It is perhaps the only single supplement we know of that can prevent deterioration of the cartilage and even repair it. None of the medicines available do that—they all "work" by relieving symptoms.

If you already have knee pain from arthritis, this should be the first treatment you use. I recommend taking 1,500 mg daily—1,000 mg in the morning and 500 mg in the evening.

There is no evidence that young adults benefit from glucosamine. But by the time you are in your thirties, you should consider taking it preventatively. Early cartilage loss is usually 100 percent reversible; at those first stages, the cartilage is not really lost, just dried out, and glucosamine can add moisture back in—and keep it there. Glucosamine on its own will do you good, but most often it is sold combined with chondroitin, which is a helpful but not required addition.

Chondroitin, a carbohydrate, is a raw material used for healthy cartilage synthesis. Like glucosamine, which it is most often used in conjunction with, it relieves joint pain, inflammation and tenderness, and restores functionality. Chondroitin also contributes to cartilage stability and strength.

Chondroitin is a very large molecule that may not be biologically available to get into the joints, so it doesn't work in an obvious way. One theory explaining its effectiveness is that your body actually creates a positive immune response to chondroitin that helps heal the cartilage—sort of the opposite of the autoimmune response that damages cartilage.

Ella, whom I introduced in Chapter Two to show how this program allowed her to stave off knee surgery for years (during which she was pain-free) and then make a record recovery after surgery, is one example of the power of glucosamine and chondroitin in action. Within twelve weeks of starting the supplements (as well as an exercise program and eating plan), her knee pain was gone.

Chondroitin should always be taken along with glucosamine, and, in fact, is almost always sold in that combination. The specific amount of chondroitin is less important than getting a good dose of glucosamine, so once you've found a capsule you like on that score, you can assume the amount of chondroitin included is sufficient. Very low levels are enough to create the immune response.

Essential Fatty Acids (EFAs)

OMEGA-3 ESSENTIAL FATTY ACIDS

Most Americans don't get enough of these healthy oils, as they are largely absent from the standard American diet (which is, not for nothing, abbreviated "SAD"). And they are called "essential" because your body doesn't manufacture them, so you must get them from outside sources. They are so important to reducing inflammation and pain that you should make every effort to get plenty of them. You can get enough in your diet for preventative purposes, mainly through fish and flax seeds, but to treat existing knee pain I recommend using supplements as well.

Fish oils are the classic source of omega-3 EFAs, with **EPA** (eicosapentaenoic acid) being the key variety found there. **DHA** (docasahexaenoic acid), which also comes from fish, runs a distant second in importance as far as the knees are concerned. You almost always find both in any pill, so the total number amount of EFAs is usually given on the label, and you should be aiming for 1,000 to 3,000 mg.

Flax seeds, another key source of omega-3s, are beneficial to the knees in large part because of the **ALA** (alpha-linolenic acid) they contain. ALA is not efficiently converted to EPA or DHA, so I don't think it should be used as your only omega-3 source.

Omega-6 EFAs, including **GLA** (gamma-linolenic acid) (which is converted into D-gamma linolenic acid in the body) also prevents and reverses inflammation, swelling and pain in the joints. Borage seed oil is the most concentrated source of GLA. You can also find it in evening primrose oil, which contains **linoleic acid** as well. As with omega-3s, you can get enough omega-6s in your diet to prevent knee problems; but if you need to *treat* them, you should use supplements. Most Americans have diets very high in omega 6s, but most of the sources are processed and contaminated so as not to be of high enough quality to even really count.

Other Supplements

There are a range of other options that have been helpful to many people with knee pain and might also work for you. You should begin with the basic guidelines laid out in the boxes in this chapter for preventing knee pain, treating early to mild knee pain, or treating mild to moderate knee pain, then pick and choose among the options described to find the ones most applicable to you if you feel you still need to do more. You should add one at a time so you can determine what actually works for you.

Many claims are made for **MSM** (Methylsulfonylmethane), but its main use has been for rheumatoid arthritis. It is found naturally in most plants and animals, including humans. It helps in stopping the inflammation process, and benefits bone and cartilage. It is, for example, a source of sulfur, which is required for cartilage growth. While supplements of MSM help synthesize certain amino acids and have antioxidant properties, exactly how it helps relieve pain from osteoarthritis is not well understood. Limited research has been done, and we could use more to pinpoint its benefits. Consider, however, that it is thought to help people with rheumatoid arthritis because the disease is inflammatory. With the latest thinking being that OA is inflammatory in nature as well, MSM becomes a good choice in those cases too.

Since cartilage is composed mainly of water and collagens, taking **collagen-forming nutrients** (amino acids and micronutrients) will give you the raw materials you need to make more cartilage. You could also take collagen directly (that's the idea of shark cartilage), but I'm skeptical about its ability to be useful after being digested. I place much more emphasis on getting the nutrients you need to let your body build its own cartilage, including the **calcium, magnesium, mucopolysaccharides, copper** (without which two collagen molecules can't stick together), **zinc** and trace minerals discussed in this chapter. You also need **protein,** which is made from amino acids. There is more protein found in collagen than in any other structure within the human body.

Amino acids—the building blocks of protein—are key components for making and repairing cartilage. If you get high-quality protein in your diet, you probably get enough, although supplements won't hurt. But if you are one of the growing fraction of Americans who eat poor-quality (processed/genetically modified/nonorganic) protein, or eat protein only at one meal a day, you should probably use supplements. Try adding some amino-acid–rich protein powder to a fruit shake or oatmeal, for example—breakfast commonly being a low-protein meal. (Additional amino acids that have specific benefits to your cartilage, immune system and muscles are included in several places in the rest of this chapter; you can recognize them by their names, which all begin with the prefix "L-," as in "L-lysine.")

SAMe (S-adenosyl-L-methionine) relieves knee pain from osteoarthritis, according to the U.S. Agency for Healthcare Research and Quality's analysis of a slate of studies that met their quality criteria. SAMe, an anti-inflammatory, may be better known for fighting depression, as studies show it not only outperforms placebos but also equals the performance of antidepressants—and with fewer side effects. But SAMe also works as well on knees as NSAIDs do, with fewer gastrointestinal side effects. (SAMe also has antidepressant properties; so as an added benefit, it may work to reinterpret pain signals in your brain, the way antidepressant drugs can.)

Capsaicin, used topically, combats pain. Studies showing that it works better than a placebo have been enough for these creams to edge into use in conventional medicine. The hot-pepper extract decreases inflammation and diminishes the number of neurotransmitters (substance P) carrying pain messages. Like other topical analgesics, capsaicin cream increases blood flow, and hence oxygen, to the affected area, creating a sensation (in this case, heat) so strong as to interfere with your body's interpretation of pain from other sources. Using this cream can increase the effectiveness of NSAIDs such as ibuprofen.

Emu oil has a long history in Australia as a topical anti-inflammatory; aboriginals and early white settlers rubbed it on to relieve joint and muscle pain (and to help heal wounds). Perhaps the antioxidants it contains are the secret of its anti-inflammatory success, or the alpha-linolenic acid and triglycerides. Some studies of arthritic rats who were anointed with emu oil showed they received pain relief equal to that of aspirin.

Silica, mucopolysaccharides and **hydroxyproline** are used in the body in forming cartilage, and are useful ingredients if you find them in combination with other nutrients you take.

Herbs

In recovering from my knee injury, one of the things I did was to take a combination of herbs to clean away metabolic debris after each workout I did. One of my colleagues, a nutritionist and a marathoner, tried the same approach after a race this fall, and told me he woke up the next morning with virtually no pain for the first time ever in the twenty or so marathons he had run. (For the record, it was a combination of just a few capsules containing antioxidants, vitamins and micronutrients such as those mentioned in this chapter, along with molybdenum, choline, parotid tissue, L-methionine, N-acetyl-L-cysteine, taurine, L-glutathione, quercetin, and the herbs red clover, boldo, burdock root, culvers root, and Joe Pye.)

That's just one way herbs are useful. They can also reduce inflammation, and stimulate repair of various kinds of tissue. There are entire books devoted to the potential of herbs, so I'm not going to go into great detail here.

The rest of this chapter provides some guidance as to how to look for the right supplements for you. There are so many combinations and formulations at so many different doses out there that you would never find an exact match for any specific recommendation I could make. Your best bet is to find one or preferably two combination products— formulated for knees or joints, most likely, or for fighting inflammation—containing many of the herbs I describe in this chapter. (If you use two different formulas, you'll get exposed to a wider array of herbs; they may overlap a few ingredients, but then each should have a list of ingredients the other doesn't contain.) Beyond that, you might also benefit from working with a professional to tailor a prescription just for you.

Here are several of the herbs that can be beneficial to the knee (most are anti-inflammatory):

Ginger, bromelain, boswellia, cayenne, cumin, and **horsetail** relieve pain and are anti-inflammatory. You may also find **devil's claw, willow bark extract, white willow, chamomile, dandelion, butcher's broom,** and **feverfew** to be helpful.

Herbs used to decrease inflammation and improve immune function, among other effects, include **green tea, slippery elm** and **kamut** (both of which can also be prepared as a tea), **hawthorn, bladder wrack algae, astragalus** and **rosemary.**

Taking herbs with powerful antioxidants such as quercetin and bioflavonoids interrupts the inflammatory cycle and protects tissues. Herbs are generally meant to be used as treatment rather than prevention. Look for high-quality, reliable products (see the box at the end of this chapter), and follow package directions for dosing. Don't overlook herbal teas (such as chamomile and ginger), and don't forget you can simply include the relevant herbs in your cooking. The curcumin in **turmeric,** which gives it its bright yellow color, is anti-inflammatory, for example, so one tasty approach is to include plenty of curried foods in your diet. (There are plenty of books about food as medicine, and herbs as food too, if you want to know more.)

Proteolytic Enzymes

I recommend digestive enzymes to many of my patients (see Chapter Five, as they help break down food to make the nutrients therein more readily accessible for your body. To those who are recovering from a serious injury or surgery, or who are dealing with a lot of swelling in their knees, I recommend adding proteolytic enzymes as well. Proteolytic enzymes digest debris, clearing it away from your body, and help with healing. Look for a combination product that includes, usually along with several herbs, many of the following: **bromelain, papain, lipase, trypsin, chymotrypsin** and **amylase.** Use according to package directions, taking it with or after food and using larger amounts with larger meals and smaller amounts with smaller meals.

Natural Therapies

There are a handful of other options available at medical centers, spas and health food stores that may be helpful.

You might also want to try a mineral-rich **mud pack.** The mainstream *Journal of Clinical Rheumatology* published a double-blind study showing that natural mud compresses provided at least temporary relief of osteoarthritis pain in the knee. After having Dead Sea mud applied five times a week for three weeks, nearly three-quarters of patients reported improvement over three months, as against about a third of the control group. The control group received mud packs devoid of the minerals found in natural mud such as the Dead Sea mud, which is rich in magnesium, calcium, potassium, chloride, sodium and other salts, proving that it is the absorption of those minerals that is important, not just the heat of the treatment.

You could reasonably expect similar results with **mineral or herb baths** ("balneotherapy," for those who like big words). **Paraffin baths** can be a useful way to take advantage of the relief heat brings, though they don't have the added benefit of delivering extra nutrients.

Massage is another useful—and often enjoyable—pain reliever, not to mention a wonderful stress reducer. I wouldn't recommend it as your sole approach to knee pain, but it can relax muscles, reroute nerve communication, improve oxygenation and increase blood flow to help in the healing process.

Mind-Body Techniques

Traditional Chinese Medicine (TCM) in general seeks not to treat symptoms but to create balance within the body as a whole. Traditionally trained practitioners wouldn't just treat you for knee pain but rather would look to restore the balance of energy in your body, the lack of which is resulting in pain. This might be done through herbs, qi gong or similar exercise, acupuncture, or other energy healing techniques—most commonly some combination thereof.

TCM holds that heartache manifests in your knee. When your

What's the Point?

In TCM and acupuncture, several energy channels are thought to be involved with knee pain, including the Leg Greater Yin (Spleen) Muscle Channel and the Leg Absolute Yin (Liver) Muscle Channel. Injuries to tendons, ligaments or cartilage in the knee (as opposed to arthritis) may be treated at acupuncture points S-35 (Xiyan), B-54 (Weizhong), and any tender spots, probably for ten to fifteen treatments. The earlier in the pain process treatment begins, the more quickly and easily you'll find relief.

---

knees hurt, you should look to your heart—your emotions—to see if you can find the true source of your pain.

Like many complementary therapies, research on TCM that follows strict mainstream medicine guidelines is hard to find, but **acupuncture,** at least, has been scientifically studied well enough for conventional groups like the Nineteenth Congress of the International League Against Rheumatism. Taking a study presented there in 1997 as an example, there is some good evidence that acupuncture can relieve knee pain due to osteoarthritis. In that study, patients who added acupuncture to their usual drug treatment twice a week for eight weeks had significantly improved pain levels compared to a group which simply continued with their usual medications and had no change in their pain over the same time frame. Patients receiving acupuncture also were better able to continue daily activities without interference due to knee pain, and the effect lasted even after acupuncture stopped (though the study followed them only for one additional month).

Melissa

I happened to see Melissa as she came in for an appointment with Dr. Sun Fook Ka, a wonderful doctor of Traditional Chinese Medicine who shares my office space. As my colleague stepped into the hallway to meet her, he took one look, from at least thirty feet away, and asked, "What's wrong with your knee?" They'd never spoken about this before, and he didn't know the purpose of her appointment. She did not walk with a limp. He simply read her energy pattern.

Melissa was in her mid-twenties, and had been struggling with knee pain for years. When my colleague examined her, he found, like a slew of doctors before him, nothing specifically wrong with her knee physiologically. Unlike the experts Melissa had consulted before, however, he didn't really expect to. According to the principles of Eastern medicine, what is happening in the knee represents what is happening in the heart. His diagnosis of Melissa: heartache. He told her she was holding on to some old heartbreak that she would have to let go.

"It was like a slap in the face when he said that," Melissa says. "My jaw just dropped. All I could think was, how did you know? And, why didn't I think of that?"

Melissa had ended a romantic relationship some years before. Since then she hadn't been able to form a successful relationship—and her knee had hurt. "Once I realized what I was holding on to, I was able to let it go," Melissa says. "The pain stopped immediately."

Melissa had one TCM treatment, but with the acceptance of the fact that she can create and resolve conflict and pain—that she held the power—she walked out of the office that day healed.

Reflexology correlates specific points on the soles of the feet to the knee (and every other part of the body, for that matter). Some practitioners also use points on the ears and hands, but the feet are usually the main focal point. Manual stimulation of the points is thought to relieve stress and tension, improve blood supply, unblock nerve impulses and restore balance in the body. But as in other holistic practices, the whole body must be considered in total. An example would be a knee problem secondary to poor digestion—the knee wouldn't improve unless the digestive organ points on the foot were also treated.

Energetic healing from a variety of traditions provides an interesting way of regarding knee pain: The knee represents the type of emotions a person is having. Your dominant leg (the right leg for right-handed people) leads the way, stepping you into the future and managing any change of direction. Your nondominant leg supports your life's decisions in the past, grounds you, connects you to your own history, and provides stability. If you are insecure about the future, it will be your dominant leg that hurts or gets injured. If you are afraid to let go of something from the past, it will be your nondominant leg.

This argument comes in several variations, depending on which school of energetic healing is in question. For example, a European energetic healing tradition holds that if you are right handed and your right knee hurts, it indicates that you are holding too much up. If your left knee hurts, it is because you are not kneeling down before God, or forces greater than yourself—you are not accepting the reality of the universe.

Furthermore, in some schools of thought the right leg represents the masculine self and the left leg the feminine.

There are many, many forms of energy healing, and emotions are only one factor that they deal with. I am giving only a few examples of how energy healing can help recognize the way in which we manifest emotions, and break negative patterns of doing so. So you should know that there is much more to energy healing. I have seen some wonderful results from a variety of types of energy healers, so if these approaches appeal to you, I encourage you to look into what is available and try what interests you.

Finding Quality Supplements

The form and the source of the supplements you use are key to the benefits you reap. You have to go the extra mile to distinguish the highest quality from the pale imitations. Buy the highest quality you can find, using the guidelines in this section. Now is not the time to shop solely for price. Be aware that at big chain stores, huge catalog companies, or any place else where huge volume allows for a low price point, quality is very likely to be low on the priority list, at least as compared to maintaining good profit margins while still keeping prices down. I've watched far too many patients come in complaining that they've been taking supplements for months or years, and nothing's worked—only to find out they've been using cheap stuff that may never have been produced for reliable efficacy and, in any case, has probably been sitting around far too long in warehouses and on store shelves to maintain whatever effectiveness it had to begin with.

You can begin by asking your doctors and other health-care professionals if they have looked into the subject and can make specific recommendations for you. Many are knowledgeable on the subject, and I hope you have one who is—or can find one.

You can make a point of using well-established brands, though off brands might be perfectly fine, and a well-known name isn't by itself a guarantee of quality.

I hope the FDA or some other reputable scientific agency will one day soon step in to provide some regulation and guidance of supplements that will allow consumers to be informed and confident about exactly what they are buying. Until that day comes, you can look for companies making "pharmaceutical grade" supplements in "FDA registered" facilities. That means the FDA has rated them as living up to the same standards of cleanliness, quality assurance and production technique that pharmaceutical companies must use. If you don't see anything noted on a product or accompanying marketing materials about that, you can call the company directly and inquire.

Another option is to look for companies that voluntarily get evaluated by the International Nutraceutical Association (INA). You can look for their seal on products, and call companies directly to ask if they have been evaluated and, if so, what the results were.

An excellent approach is to obtain independent evaluations of specific products. The subscription website ConsumerLab.com, for example, evaluates many vitamins, herbs and other supplements for potency and purity, among other key points. You can search the website for free, and if they have evaluated the product you are looking into, it may well be worth paying the fee for the complete information. They also license a flask-shaped "seal of approval" to products that meet their standards, so seeing one on a product label should bring you some peace of mind.

This isn't just about idle curiosity. When Canadian researchers checked the amount of active ingredient in fourteen different glucosamine products, they found an actual content ranging from 300 mg to 150 mg—though eleven of them were labeled as containing 500 mg. Without knowing how reliable a product is, it is hard to ensure not only that you get the appropriate dose, but also that the activity of the product is good.

What's in a "Good" Multi?

To give you something to compare labels against, here is what I recommend in a multivitamin and mineral supplement. This is a "wish list," and you're never going to find a perfect match. And that is OK! The precise combinations and ratios of nutrients you get are not critical. Whatever combinations you look at may well have a range of things in them not mentioned here, and that too is fine. With so many permutations of multivitamins out there, there is no one perfect multivitamin for everyone. Try to find one that has the majority of the nutrients you are looking for in it.

Most of the dosages here are many times higher than just the "recommended daily value" for any given nutrient. That's because those daily values (RDA) are set to prevent deficiency, meaning they are far less than what would be ideal amounts for your body to have available for optimum health, and certainly below what's necessary to fight health problems.

If the thought of poring over all those labels down a long, long aisle in the store overwhelms you, here's a helpful shortcut: Look for a good quality multi with minerals that has at least 50 mg of the B vitamins.

If it meets that standard, in all probability it has sufficient amounts of its other ingredients.

AMOUNT PER DAY:

- Vitamin A: 15,000 IU (5,000 or less as palmitate and the remainder as beta-carotene)
- Vitamin C: 250–1,000 mg
- Vitamin D: 400 IU (D_3 would be my preference)
- Vitamin E: (as D-alpha tocopherol succinate): 150 IU, plus about 250 IU additional of mixed tocopherols and tocotrienols
- Thiamin: 75 mg
- Riboflavin: 75 mg
- Niacin (as niacinamide): 75 mg
- Vitamin B_6: 75 mg
- Folic Acid: 400 mcg
- Vitamin B_{12}: 75–1,000 mcg
- Biotin: 75 mcg
- Pantothenic Acid (B_5): 75mg
- Calcium: 20–1,000 mg
- Iodine (from kelp): 150 mcg
- Magnesium: 10 mg (or about half as much as calcium taken)
- Zinc: 10–25 mg
- Selenium: 25–200 mcg
- Copper: 1 mg
- Manganese: 1–10 mg
- Chromium: 25–300 mcg
- Potassium: 1.8 mg
- Boron: 0.5 mg (or more)

BASIC SUPPLEMENTS FOR PREVENTING AND TREATING KNEE PAIN

For generally healthy adults with a reasonably good (but not necessarily perfect) diet aiming to prevent knee pain, I recommend the following basic supplements (with daily doses):

Glucosamine: 1,500 mg (1,000 mg in the morning and 500 in the evening)

Chondroitin: Whatever amount comes with the glucosamine you choose, probably in the range of 150 to 1,500 mg

Omega-3 and omega-6 essential fatty acids: 1,000 to 3,000 mg of each, depending on how much you get in your diet. Most people should take equal amounts of omega-3s and omega-6s. Be sure your supplement includes the different types of omega-3s.

Multivitamin: Take a good quality multi with minerals that has at least 50 mg of the B vitamins, and the majority of the nutrients you are looking for.

Antioxidants: Take a well-rounded combination as directed on the bottle.

Vitamin E: 400 to 800 IU mixed tocopherols and tocotrienols. (Count whatever you get in a multivitamin and an antioxidant combination toward your dose; the total from all sources should be up to about 800.)

Calcium: 1,200 to 1,500 mg, depending on how much you get in your diet

Vitamin D: At least 800 mg, representing plenty of D_3

Magnesium: 600 to 1,000 mg; at least half of the amount of calcium you take

Trace minerals including boron, selenium, manganese, zinc and copper, plus vitamin K and probably more minerals. You should be able to get these in combination with calcium, magnesium and vitamin D.

Note: This regimen is designed to be used along with all the other approaches in this book, including eating right, getting good exercise, reducing stress and connecting your mind and body.

BASIC SUPPLEMENTS FOR EARLY OR MILD KNEE PAIN

For early or mild recurrent problems with knee pain, I recommend everything outlined in the basic plan for preventing knee pain, above, with the addition of 20 to 100 mg of some or all of the following: **L-lysine, L-proline, hawthorn, horsetail, bromelain, protease, turmetric, rosemary** and **bladderwrack algae**. As long as you use a quality product, the exact combination and dosage don't matter. Look for a combination supplement labeled for knee or joint pain—it is likely to contain most (if not all) of these ingredients. Take it according to the package directions. Use this full range for 12 to 20 weeks, until you've experienced relief that has lasted for a while, then scale back to the basic prevention plan.

BASIC SUPPLEMENTS FOR MILD TO MODERATE KNEE PAIN

If you have additional symptoms, such as swelling, stiffness and pain, or your symptoms are more intense or have lasted longer, add to the two plans above a combination of 10 to 100 mg of some or all of the following: **molybdenum, L-methionine, choline, taurine, L-glutathione, quercetin, papain, lipase, amylase, trypsin, chymotrypsin, SOD** and **catalase**. Look for a combination supplement, probably one labeled for knee or joint pain, that contains most (if not all) of these ingredients. Take it according to the package directions. Once you get relief, cut back to the second level plan for twelve weeks. If you still have no symptoms, then cut back to the basic plan.

If you haven't found some benefit by six to twelve weeks on this program, you should consult a holistic health-care professional to better personalize a plan for you. For moderate to severe pain, you should seek out the assistance of a holistic health-care practitioner from the start.

NUTRIENTS FOR THYROID HORMONE HEALTH

Look for combination products (often sold as thyroid formulas) with a good range of the following nutrients to help keep your thyroid levels healthy:

- Vitamin A
- Vitamin D
- Vitamin C
- Vitamin E
- Niacinamide
- Riboflavin
- Zinc
- *Withania somnifera* (ashwagandha)
- Selenium
- Guggals
- Chromium
- Cadmium
- Copper
- Omega-3 essential fatty acids (especially DHA, EPA and CLA)
- Carnosic acid

Note: Some supplements, medications and foods can interfere with thyroid function. So pay attention to your intake of **homocystine, alpha lipoic acid, L-carnitine, cortisol**, and **soy**. Homocystine lowers thyroid function. At high doses, lipoic acid (over 1,000 mg) and L-carnitine (2,000 to 4,000 mg or more) decrease T3 by decreasing the change of T4 into T3. Cortisol increases reverse T3, and therefore also decrease T3. Soy, if you get 25 to 45 grams or more each day, decreases absorption of thyroid hormones.

NUTRIENTS FOR HORMONE BALANCE

Look for combination products with a good range of the following nutrients to help you balance your hormones:

- Vitamin A
- Vitamin D
- Vitamin C
- Vitamin B_5
- Vitamin B_6
- Taurine
- Bio soy flavonoids (such as kudzu)
- Lignans (found in flax seeds)
- I3C (indol-3-carbonol)
- DIM (diindolylmethane)
- EFAs (essential fatty acids)

10

Keep On Moving

Exercise will help you live longer, move better, sleep better, have more energy, improve your mood and build your self-confidence to boot. Plus, it's all natural! And inexpensive! If I said all that about any given medicine, you'd think I was a snake oil salesman, but this is all well established in the mainstream medical literature.

Now I'd like to help you take advantage of one more benefit of exercise: avoiding or eliminating knee pain. Anyone can do this quick and easy workout, which is specifically designed to protect and strengthen your knee. All you need is a simple set of ankle weights, inexpensive exercise rubber bands and just minutes a day.

You should experience relief from your knee pain within six to eight weeks, using these exercises in conjunction with proper nutrition and the other techniques covered in this book, assuming your problem is a mild to moderate one. Three months will do it for 90 percent of the most usual knee problems, including "bad knees," old injuries, and post-surgery recovery. (In the wake of a knee injury or surgery, you'll need physical therapy geared specially to you.)

For those of you with no knee pain, these exercises will help you keep it that way!

For pain-free knees, you need balanced muscle tone and balanced muscle utilization—and sound balance—which is just what these techniques deliver. You need exercises that work on strength, balance, range of motion, coordination and flexibility, which this program is designed to do. You need to make sure your quads and hamstrings have proportionate strength, that both legs are equally strong, that your various quadriceps muscles (there are actually four) have properly distributed strength, and that your gluteal muscles are strong so they work in concert with the quads, all of which this program ensures. Balanced strength and coordination promotes joint stability and prevents injuries.

The workout in this chapter comes in three phases. The first phase consists of a series of five exercises done with ankle weights. The movements are what physical therapists would consider "open-chain" (as opposed to "closed-chain") exercises, because of the way resistance is used and the way muscles and joints are worked. Open-chain exercises generally isolate muscles and produce stronger muscle contractions. Closed-chain exercises generally involve groups of muscles, more closely approximating the way muscles are used in real-life activities.

Even among health-care professionals, however, there's significant debate over the fine points of what exactly "open chain" and "closed chain" consist of, and which are better under what circumstances. I don't want to belabor the point here because in the end, a combination is what you're going to want. But since you may hear the terms bandied about, I thought you should know how the workout here would be classified, and how I developed its phases.

More useful, in my opinion, is to think in terms of "functional," or "skill," training, which aims not only to strengthen muscles but also to improve coordination, flexibility and balance, to get you ready to do all the subtly complex movements of everyday life. Officially, closed-chain exercises are functional, though in point of fact, both open- and closed-chain exercises can be functional, and any given function may require both open- and closed-chain movements. Often functional, or skill, training is used to mean sports-specific exercises (i.e., what hurdlers need differs from what speed skaters need differs from what you need for twice weekly beginners' yoga classes). But I like to think of the combination program presented here as an example of real functional training in that it is all you need to function well through whatever you do in the course of your day.

The second phase of my program, then, is five closed-chain exercises done mainly with exercise rubber bands. The third phase incorporates machines found at most gyms, for those of you who want to take advantage of that membership, though in terms of overall results it is strictly optional. Using machines is not necessary for healthy knees, and these exercises are not necessarily better than the at-home techniques. They can, however, add interest and variety to your program, as well as different kinds of challenges for your muscles. When and if you are ready to move on to machines—when you know your muscles are capable of doing more work and your knee feels stable and strong, and you have built up the amount of resistance you work with and feel you could increase the reps—you can phase out Phase One.

Do your complete workout at least three or four times each week, or do at least a few exercises each day (for example, one phase one day, and another the next). You should begin with Phase One, performing that series of exercises until you can do all of them with reasonable ease, having worked up to six to eight pounds or more in your ankle weights. Add in Phase Two at that point. You can probably complete both phases in about twenty minutes using proper form.

But do not rush, or you will sacrifice form—and so, both effectiveness and safety. Slow and steady movement is always better. It gives your muscles a chance to adjust, your joints a chance to stabilize as you go along, and your muscles and brain time to communicate and provide feedback. Working against whatever amount of resistance challenges your muscles yet allows you to maintain good form is the only way to build proper strength and function of related muscles.

This is a regimen that any generally healthy person with a knee problem, or concerned about developing a knee problem, could do and benefit from. It is aimed at resolving most mild to moderate, slowly advancing knee pain. *Anyone with a serious medical condition should consult with a medical professional before beginning an exercise program of any kind. This program is NOT for anyone with a red, hot, swollen knee and fever, or anyone who had a sudden onset of intense knee pain for no apparent reason. In any case, if you've never worked with weights before, or never been instructed on how to do so safely and efficiently, you may want to start with a supervised workout.*

Ideally, you'd get an individualized exercise prescription customized to your specific circumstances, though obviously that is impossible in a book. What I've provided here is a good, solid way to get just about anyone started. In addition to the exercises described here, and the aerobic exercise you need for overall good health, you should also be sure to strengthen the rest of your body, and especially your "core"—your abs, obliques, and lower back muscles. (You can do this with the appropriate equipment at any gym; with a Pilates class, book or videotape; working with a physical therapist or an experienced trainer; or even with calisthenics-type exercises—old fashioned sit-ups, crunches and so on.)

As you continue with any exercise program, over time you'll gradually be able to do more, or do more intense exercise, and so you will progress in how much resistance you use in these exercises. Just remember, the goal isn't to move as much weight as possible but to move whatever weight you can in such a way as to maximize function, strength and stability. Good form is paramount in effectiveness and efficiency, as well as safety. Any exercise you do should be just intense enough to fatigue the muscles you are working on. Your program should never exhaust you.

Doing this workout will point out your existing weaknesses to you. You may, for example, be stronger on one side than the other, or better at one exercise than another. I've had strong patients, regular exercisers, who'd try a simple exercise requiring balance and have to grab for a chair so as not to fall over. Clearly, their bodies are fit, but not functioning well. No wonder their knees hurt.

Throughout this program, it is important to strengthen both sides of your body. That is, work both knees, not just the "bad" one. And use the same weight on both sides, even if that means one leg moves less than it could at first. Stick with whatever the "bad" knee can handle, on both sides. For one thing, your weaker leg will improve much faster if you work out both legs. But more important is ensuring symmetrical strength, as well as supporting your nerves and muscles in coordinating movements smoothly.

You should also remember that in many of the exercises, the leg you are standing on is getting just as important a workout as the one you are moving. Standing on one leg as you lift weight with the other, for example, helps the body learn to shift and balance, and the brain to talk to the muscles on both sides of the body at once. This is exactly what we mean when we are talking about proprioception. It is not just about lifting a weight; it is about reprogramming your body and your brain into positive patterns of movement.

Warm up before you begin. Do at least five minutes walking or on a stationary bike—until your body feels physically warm (there is no exact length of time that takes, and it will depend in large part on how fast you are walking or riding). If you ride, be sure to set the bike seat high enough (your leg should extend fully—with your knee straight—when you sit on the seat and place your heel on the pedal at the bottom of its arc) to reduce force on the knee. The last few inches of knee straightening can be up to 40 percent of the benefit you receive. If you use a treadmill, do a slow walk, without any incline, to warm up. Despite long-standing advice, stretching before a workout has no effect on reducing pain, but stretching *afterward*, especially your quads and hamstrings, is a very good idea.

Phase One

You'll need a set of ankle weights for this phase, the kind that wrap around your ankle and fasten with Velcro, with pockets for 1- to 2-pound weights all around them. Keep weights on both ankles for the entire exercise set. Begin this phase using 2 pounds on each ankle. If this is too intense, begin with weights on your thigh above your knee. For each rep of the exercise, count to 3 as you perform the first part of the move, hold for a count of 5, and return to start for a count of 5. Lowering your leg may be even more important than raising it, so take your time; move slowly. The point is to use the muscle correctly, not to simply lift the weight.

Perform each exercise 15 times per set, rest for 30 seconds (and not longer than a minute) between sets, then repeat another set before going on to the other side. The last few reps in each set should be a little difficult, and you should need that rest in order to have your muscles "catch their breath" and do the next set properly. As your strength increases, and the last few reps are no longer particularly difficult, increase the amount of weight you are using by 2 pounds. Once you are up to 6 or 8 pounds, as I mentioned, you should begin to add Phase Two to your workout.

Whatever amount of weight you are using, these exercises should never be so hard to do that you strain while doing them. They are designed to isolate particular leg muscles, and should never be so difficult that you have to squeeze your neck or stomach or back muscles. You want the targeted muscles to be strong enough to do the work on their

Breathe

To help you lift the weight up, let your breath out as you do so, starting just before you begin lifting and continuing all the way through the lift.

own (this is, after all, why you are doing the program). Focus your mind (thinking good thoughts!) on the muscles the exercise targets, and try to relax the others.

You should also be sure to maintain good body alignment while you perform these exercises, just as with any other activity. It's a good general habit, but it is also another way to protect your knees, as well as train the muscles properly. Watch in particular that you don't arch your lower back.

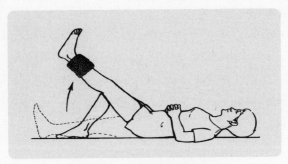

Used with permission from the Saunders Group, Inc.

• *Leg raise, front* •

(FOR YOUR ANTERIOR QUADS)

Lie on your back with right knee bent at about 90 degrees and the right foot placed flat on the floor, and the left leg, with an ankle weight, extended straight out along the floor. Slowly and steadily—for the count of 3—raise your left leg, keeping it completely straight—but not locked—until your leg is at a 30- to 45-degree angle. Hold for a count of 5, then lower your leg back down to the floor for another count of 5. Do 2 sets of 15 repetitions. Complete both sets, then switch sides.

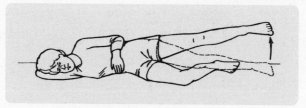

Used with permission from the Saunders Group, Inc.

• *Side leg raise #1* •

(FOR YOUR LATERAL QUADS AND HIP ABDUCTORS)

Lie on your right side, with your head resting on your bent right elbow for support, your hips aligned one on top of the other. For stability, bend your right leg slightly, and place your left hand flat on the floor a few inches in front of your waist or rest it lightly on your waist. Keeping both knees facing forward (the same way your face is facing), raise your left leg straight up toward the ceiling until it is at a 30- to 45-degree angle. Keep it in line with your right leg; do not let it come forward. Hold, then lower it to the start position. Perform 15 repetitions. Complete your first set; then do side leg raise #2 on the same side before rolling over to your left side to do 1 set of both exercises.

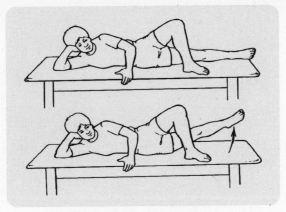

Used with permission from the Saunders Group, Inc.

• *Side leg raise #2* •

(FOR YOUR MEDIAL QUADS AND HIP ADDUCTORS)

Lie on your right side with your head propped up on your right arm
(bent at the elbow) and your left hand flat on the floor a few inches in
front of your waist to stabilize you. Bend your left leg to place your foot
flat on the floor in front of your right knee. Raise your right leg toward
the ceiling, keeping the knee and toes facing forward (the same way your
face is facing), until it is at a 30- to 45-degree angle. Hold, and return to
start. Do 15 repetitions. Complete side leg raise #1 and #2 on one side,
then roll to your other side and perform both exercises on the other leg.
(When you finish your second set of side leg raises #1 and #2 lying on
your right side, roll onto your left side and do your second set of both
exercises on that side.)

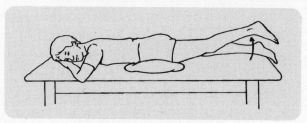

Used with permission from the Saunders Group, Inc.

• *Leg raise, backward* •
(FOR YOUR GLUTEALS AND HAMSTRINGS)

Lie on your belly with your head turned to one side, resting on your hands. If you experience discomfort in your lower back with this exercise, try placing a small pillow under your waist. Raise your left leg off the floor, bending only at the hip, until it is at an angle of 30 to 45 degrees or as high as you can comfortably go, hold, and return to start. Complete 2 sets of 15 reps each, then do the right leg. You may find that it takes a while to build up to that amount of extension (30 to 45 degrees) with your leg, but don't push it; build up to it gradually.

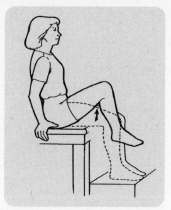

Used with permission from the Saunders Group, Inc.

• *Knee raise* •

(FOR YOUR QUADS AND HIP FLEXORS)

Sit securely on the front edge of a chair or bed with your knees bent at a 90-degree angle and your feet flat on the floor directly in front of you. Bending at the right hip, raise your right knee toward the ceiling until it is at a thirty- to forty-five-degree angle, hold, and return to start. Complete 2 sets of 15 reps, then do the left leg.

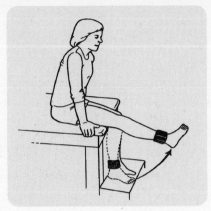

Used with permission from the Saunders Group, Inc.

• *Knee extension* •

(FOR YOUR QUADS AND HIP FLEXORS)

Once the knee raise is reasonably easy with 6 or 8 pounds of weight, switch to this more aggressive version of the exercise. Begin as above, but after your knee is lifted to thirty to forty-five degrees, straighten your leg for a count of 5 while maintaining the bend in your hip. Bend knee again and lower the leg to start for a count of 5. Complete 2 sets, then do the other leg.

Phase Two

This phase adds the challenge of balancing on one leg while working the other; this is, besides strength training, a good start on a proprioceptive workout.

For this phase, you'll need a few exercise rubber bands of different strengths, so you can start with less resistance and increase it as you get stronger. As with weights, move up to the next level of resistance when you can complete your sets with relative ease, to preserve the challenge of the exercise. For the last exercise, you'll also need a step, bench or box large and sturdy enough to hold your weight securely, and perhaps a set of light hand weights.

As before, you should do two sets of 15 reps of each exercise, resting 30 to 60 seconds between sets. Use the same counts: 3 up, pause 5, 5 down. Work up to being able to extend your leg to a forty-five-degree angle.

For each of the first four exercises here, you'll need to anchor the rubber band to or around something stationary, such as a sturdy table leg or a closed door. The other end will go around one of your ankles. You can purchase adapters that anchor the bands to your foot and to a door.

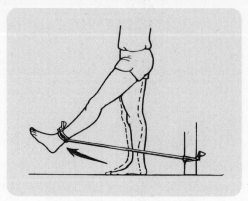

Used with permission from the Saunders Group, Inc.

• *Forward leg sweep* •

(FOR YOUR ANTERIOR QUADS)

With the rubber band around your left ankle, stand with your back to the anchoring object, far enough away that the band is just taut but not tightly stretched. While balancing your body weight on the stationary right leg, slowly raise your left leg straight out in front of you as far as you can stretch the band, hold, and return to start. Repeat on your right after 2 sets of 15 reps with the left leg.

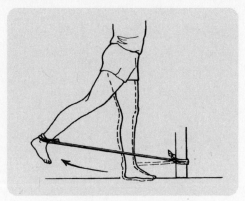

Used with permission from the Saunders Group, Inc.

• *Backward leg sweep* •

(FOR YOUR GLUTEALS AND HAMSTRINGS)

Stand facing the anchoring object with the rubber band around your right ankle and pulled taut. Raise your right leg straight back, going as far as you can stretch the band, hold, and return to the starting position. Repeat on your right after 2 sets of 15 reps.

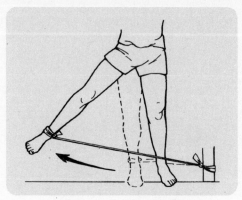

Used with permission from the Saunders Group, Inc.

• *Outside leg sweep* •

(FOR YOUR LATERAL QUADS AND HIP ABDUCTORS)

Standing with your left side toward the anchoring object and the band around your right ankle, raise your right hip and leg straight out to your right side, without letting your hip come forward, hold, and return to start. Repeat with your left leg after 2 sets of 15 reps.

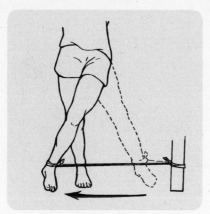

Used with permission from the Saunders Group, Inc.

• *Inside leg sweep* •

(FOR YOUR MEDIAL QUADS AND HIP ABDUCTORS)

Stand with your left side toward the anchoring object, the band around your left ankle, and the toes of your left foot pointed out to the side. Cross your left leg in front of your standing leg and lift as far as you can to the right; cross behind for half the reps. Repeat with your right leg after 2 sets.

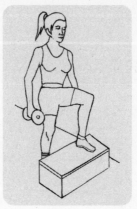

Copyright PhysioTools Ltd. Altered with permission of PhysioTools Ltd.

• *Step up* •

(FOR YOUR QUADS AND HIP FLEXORS)

Stand in front of a bench, box or step with a light hand weight in your right hand. Step up onto it, leading with your left foot, for a count of 3 to 5. Once both feet are flat on the step, step down again, leading with your left leg, again for a count of 3 to 5. Complete 2 sets of 15, then repeat, leading with your right foot. Each time your knee bends, make sure it moves out directly over your shoelaces, and doesn't angle to either side. Once you've mastered this exercise and are ready to increase the challenge, you can vary it to increase the challenge, as follows.

Stand with both feet on the step, with your left leg close to the left side of the step. Hold the weight in your left hand. Standing on your right leg, move your left foot out to the side and lower it as far down as you can go, without touching the floor, to a count of 3 to 5, and return to standing for the same count. Do 2 sets of 15, then switch to the other leg for 2 sets.

Then do the same basic motion, lowering your foot toward the floor and returning to standing, but this time with your left foot just in front of the step. After 2 sets, repeat with the left foot just behind the step.

Phase Three

When Phase Two has become much easier than it was when you started, and you feel strong, secure and balanced, then those of you who are interested in working out on machines are ready to drop Phase One exercises in favor of Phase Three. (If you don't want to move on to Phase Three, find more challenging ways to perform the basic exercises in Phases One and Two—more resistance being the most obvious way. But there are also many other exercises you can do. A physical therapist or a good trainer is your best bet for learning them, although you can also pick some up from books or videos.)

You can do many of the Phase Three exercises on a "multi-hip" machine (the first four, in fact), although at your gym you might also use the hip abductor and adductor machines. Use other machines as needed or desired. The same or very similar exercises can be done on just about any brand of machine your chosen gym stocks. If your gym doesn't have the exact machines described here, it will have something that works similar muscles, and someone there should be able to help you adapt these exercises in just a few minutes.

Whatever machine you use, be sure it is appropriately adjusted to your body—especially, for this series of exercises, to your height and leg length. That's one good thing about the multi-hip: It is infinitely adjustable, so you can get just the right proportions for you in each position you use.

As with earlier phases, do 2 sets of 15 reps of each exercise, except where noted. Once again, you should count to 3 for the initial move, hold it for 5, and take another 5 to return to the starting position. Begin with light weights, just enough to fatigue your muscles for each set; the last few reps of each set should be a little difficult. Increase your weights as you get stronger so that the last few reps of each set are a little difficult, though still doable with good form. The idea is always to fatigue, but not exhaust, your muscles.

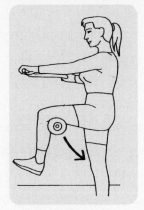

Copyright PhysioTools Ltd.

• *Standing hip extension* •

(FOR YOUR HAMSTRINGS AND HIP EXTENDERS)

Stand with your right side toward the multi-hip machine and raise your left leg over the roller, which should be about 90 degrees in front of you. Hold on to the support bar for stability. Keep your upper body still, and extend your left leg backward by tightening your buttock muscles. You should be able to swing your leg 45 degrees backward and 90 degrees forward with each repetition of this exercise.

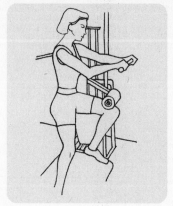

Copyright PhysioTools Ltd. Altered with permission of PhysioTools Ltd.

• *Standing hip flexion* •

(FOR YOUR QUADS AND HIP FLEXORS)

Here, instead of 2 sets of 15 of the same exercise, you'll do 3 sets of 10—1 set each of 3 different variations on the exercise—before switching to work the other leg. You can work up to 2 sets of 10 of each part if you wish.

Part One: Stand with your left side toward the multi-hip machine with your left thigh under the roller. Hold the support bar and keep your upper body still. Lift your left thigh and knee until your hip bends to a 90-degree angle. Holding your hip there, extend your leg for a count of 3, hold for 5, and then bend it, again, slowly, keeping your hip high. Do this 10 times, then lower your hip back to standing.

Part Two: Begin as in Part One. Raise your hip the same way, hold for a count of 5, and return to standing. (You are omitting the leg extension of Part One.) Do this 9 more times.

Part Three: The movement is the same as Part Two except you turn your hip and knee out, so that your inner thigh muscles are doing the work. Do 1 set of 10.

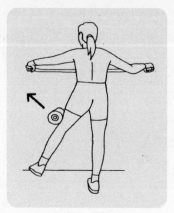

Copyright PhysioTools Ltd.

• *Standing hip abduction* •

(FOR YOUR LATERAL QUADS AND HIP ABDUCTORS)

Stand in front of the multi-hip machine, with the hinge level with your mid-thigh. Keeping your upper body still (you should not be using so much weight that you need to lean to move it), lift your left leg outward against the pad to 45 to 60 degrees for 3 counts, hold for 5, then lower again for 5. Do 2 sets of 15 repetitions with the left leg, then repeat with the right leg.

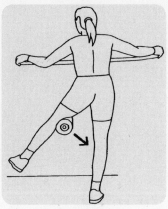

Copyright PhysioTools Ltd.

• *Standing hip adduction* •

(FOR YOUR MEDIAL QUADS AND HIP ADDUCTORS)

Stand facing the multi-hip machine. Position the roller in its upper position, against the inner left leg at mid-thigh level. Hold on to the support bar, and keep your upper body still. Pull your leg down and in toward your standing leg. Hold, then lift again, following the usual counts of 3-5-5. Do 2 sets of 15 repetitions and then switch legs.

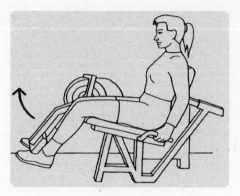

Copyright PhysioTools Ltd.

• *Seated leg extension* •

(FOR YOUR ANTERIOR QUADS)

With your ankles under the foot pads, straighten your legs with your feet in a flexed position; hold for a count of 5 and lower, for 2 sets of 15 reps. You can advance to adding 1 set of 10, using both legs to raise the weight and only one leg to lower it, and then to 1 set of 10 on each side, using one leg to raise and lower the weight.

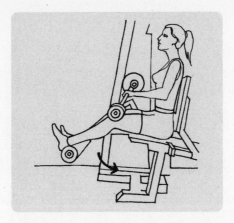

Copyright PhysioTools Ltd. Altered with permission of PhysioTools Ltd.

• *Seated leg curl* •

(FOR YOUR GLUTEALS AND HAMSTRINGS)

Sit on the leg-curl machine with your legs extended straight out in front of you, the back of your knees over the pad, and your ankles resting on the bar. Pull your lower legs down and back, toward a regular seated position, as if you were in a chair. Hold, then return to start. As in the seated leg extension, when you are ready, advance to adding 1 set of 10, using both legs to raise and only one to lower the weight, then to 1 set of 10 on each side, using just one leg at a time to raise and lower the weight.

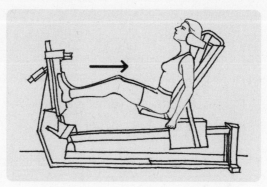

Copyright PhysioTools Ltd. Altered with permission of PhysioTools Ltd.

• *Seated leg press* •

(FOR YOUR QUADS AND HIP FLEXORS)

I've designed this exercise for the type of machine I prefer, one in which you push your body away from the foot rest rather than the foot rest away from your body. You'll see why as you follow the progressions. If your gym has the other kind of machine, you can do the same basic exercise, though you won't be able to do the final variations.

Place both feet shoulder-width apart on the foot rest. Push your body away, being sure to use both legs evenly, for a count of 5, then slowly return to start, also for a count of 5.

When you can complete both sets easily at a weight equal to at least a quarter of your body weight, then switch to this variation: Push away using both legs, but return using only one leg at a time. Complete 2 sets with the return on the same leg, then do 2 sets with the return on the other leg.

When this is easy using weights equal to at least half your body weight (having worked up to that, starting with low weights and increasing gradually to maintain just enough resistance to fatigue but not exhaust your muscles), substitute this variation: Push away with both feet and return using only one leg, with the foot placed in the middle of the foot rest. Eventually, you should work up to returning with one leg on the right side of the foot rest for 2 sets of 15 reps, and on the left side for 2 sets of 15 reps.

The next step is to push away hard enough with both legs that your feet leave the foot rest (almost like a seated jump), and land and return using only one leg, with the foot placed in the middle of the foot rest. Eventually, you should add "jumping" with both legs and returning with one leg on the right side of the foot rest for 2 sets of 15 reps, and on the left side for 2 sets of 15 reps for each leg, and then to "jumping" and landing with just one leg. Finish your sets with one leg before switching to the other leg.

Have a Ball

Several types of exercise will help prepare your knees for absorbing the impact and shock of walking, jogging, stair climbing and so on. Forms of exercise that are especially good for sore knees include exercising in water (which supports your weight, thereby taking the stress off your joints), and performing balance and coordination exercises (which improves mind-muscle communication and coordinates multiple muscle groups at one time) using balance boards, wobble boards and those large rubber exercise balls—sometimes known as gym balls, physical therapy balls, or, using a brand name generically, Physioballs. Something as simple as pointing and flexing your feet against as much resistance (meaning anything you can push against—a wall, water, an exercise band) as you can comfortably handle can help too. So can stepping onto and off of a rolled up towel, or standing on one leg while bouncing (dribbling) a ball. You can also set up a little obstacle course for yourself—then try navigating it with your hands on your hips, or while repeatedly tossing a ball.

I'm mentioning this because although these three phases should restore your knees and/or keep them healthy, they aren't the only workout that can do so. If you love this one, by all means, stick to it. But if you find yourself tiring of it, please branch out—try new things or new variations and combinations. You should actually *enjoy* exercising, doing something good for your body and your self—maybe not every single time, but overall. So find the fun in it if you can, and at the very least, take a moment to appreciate what it does for you—what you are doing for yourself.

APPENDIX

Though this is not a comprehensive list, I like these labs for saliva hormone tests:

Aeron Life Cycles Clinical Lab: 800-631-7900
Sabre Science Inc.: 888-490-7300

The following labs (again, not a comprehensive list) have a holistic orientation and offer a wide variety of testing, including assessments of digestive, immune, endocrine and metabolic function, and nutritional status:

Doctors Data Inc.: 800-323-2784
Great Smokies Diagnostic Laboratories: 800-522-4762
Metametrix Clinical Laboratories: 800-221-4640

Another not-thorough list of nutraceutical companies I like (some products are available only through health-care practitioners' offices):

Allergy Research Group   Desert Herbals
Biotics Research   Designs for Health

Douglas Laboratories

Herbal Alchemist

Metabolics

Metagenics

Nordic Naturals

Nutri-West

Pathway Inc.

Physiologics

Phyto Pharmacia

Progressive Laboratories

Pure Encapsulations

Research Nutrition

Thorn Research

Vitamin Research

Yasoo

INDEX